RN Bound

A Guide to Becoming a Successful Nurse

Yalanda D. Comeaux
MSN, M.J., RN, CMSRN

TABLE OF CONTENTS

ACKNOWLEDGMENTS

First and foremost, my biggest and most heartfelt thank you goes to my wonderful husband, Andre, who was my greatest supporter during the long, stressful hours that surrounded the writing of this book. I love and appreciate him so much for providing me endless encouragement, love, support, and faith throughout the entire process.

To all my former incredible students who came through in answering my call in being a part of my research in order to make this book possible, I want to sincerely thank you all. It is your responses, guidance, and wisdom that shall depict the reality of the nursing profession to the reader of this book. Your expert advice is most invaluable, and I very much appreciate each of you who chose to be a part of this. To those who have mentored me over the years, or have sent words of encouragement my way, I want to thank all of you from the bottom of my heart. I assure you all that you have given me the gift that continues to give.

I consistently work hard each and every day to teach and train students to guide them to being the greatest nurses possible; the kind of nurses that are the very best in providing quality care for patients. I'm so grateful to the many patients I've had the pleasure of knowing and taking care of over the years and feel blessed to have had the opportunity to touch their lives during their times of health needs.

I am grateful to be continually afforded wonderful opportunities to perform my talent in nursing and to show my compassion and experiences to others. Without those experiences, there is little doubt that I would be the nurse I am today. I truly love being a nurse, and it is my sincere hope that my passion and enthusiasm for this phenomenal profession will shine through each page.

INTRODUCTION

Ever since the beginning of the mid-19th century, students across the globe have been enrolling in nursing school in pursuit of obtaining nursing degrees and taking the extraordinary leap into becoming professional nurses. First and foremost, I must congratulate you on your career choice! Nursing is unlike any other career in the world; it's a special one. It can be found at the intersection where passion meets determination, and it is a career where it takes a very specific person to achieve success in this role. In addition, it's a position that will allow you to touch people's lives and have a long-lasting effect on them. Because of this reason (as well as many others), the nursing profession remains one of the most respected and sought after professions today, even more than doctors, lawyers, pharmacists, policemen (and policewomen), and firemen (and firewomen). If you are reading this book, it means you have already chosen to attend nursing school, or perhaps you're thinking about the idea and you're still a bit unsure whether nursing is the right career path for you. This is where this book will provide value to you.

Who am I and what qualifies me to write a book on this topic? Well ... I am a Nurse clinician, I am a Nurse educator, I am a Nurse leader, I am a Nurse mentor, and I am a Nurse advocate who fights for nursing causes and the best outcome of her patients. My background is as such. Before becoming a registered nurse I worked in the healthcare industry in some capacity. I have more than 30 years in the industry, beginning as a lab assistant. I was a pharmacy technician and a nurse's aid, all before eventually becoming a nurse. As a practicing registered nurse for 20 years and counting, I must say that there is truly no amount of training that could have prepared me for some of the things which I have seen during my tenure. You can only be trained for certain things; other things you have to experience first-hand and do the very best you can. Over the years in caring for patients, many people would comment, "I bet you have seen it all." To which I would reply, "Yeah, I could write a book," which brings me here, talking to you about the nursing field and giving you my personal perspective on the world of nursing from someone who knows the profession and isn't going to sugarcoat it for you. I'm going to keep it real!

The primary reason I felt so compelled to write this book is for the mere fact that since I have been teaching, I cannot count the number of times a student has said to me, "I wish I knew this before I enrolled because I would have been more prepared or may have possibly made a different decision about choosing nursing as a career at the least."

As you can imagine, hearing those words is never a good thing, and I never enjoy it when a student enters my class on the first day unaware of what it really takes to become a successful nurse or what nursing entails. Since this aforementioned depiction happens more often than I would like to acknowledge, it is very important that students thinking of enrolling in nursing schools are given a guide to assist them in their decision. Currently, on average, students entering the field lack the clear understanding of what it means to be a nurse, have a wrong perception of nursing, and do not have an understanding of the word "care" in nursing. These facts fueled my passion to provide this imperative information. This book will serve as a roadmap for a novice nurse, or someone who is thinking of enrolling in nursing school and currently weighing their options. It will also assist a nursing student who needs advice on how to manage and prioritize his or her schedule and most importantly, how to finally arrive at the finish

line of the National Council Licensure Examination —
NCLEX exam!

COMMON MYTHS ABOUT THE NURSING PROFESSION

Okay, so we're all aware of the fact that there are
myths surrounding nursing school. As are all myths,
these are untrue. Listed below are some common
nursing myths that still circulate. Following each myth
is the truth about the subject from none other than the
experts in the field.

MYTH: Nursing school is easy.
Truth: Nursing school is a lot of things, but easy certainly
isn't one of them. If you attend nursing school because
you've been told "it's easy," then you're in for quite the
rude awakening. Your days will be filled with classes,
lectures, and clinicals, followed by hours of studying
for examinations. As a general rule of thumb, you can
expect to study 2 hours for every 1 hour of class you
attend.

MYTH: Nurses are simply people who couldn't become
doctors.
Truth: We did not fail at becoming doctors. We chose
to be nurses. Nurses and doctors are not the same and
comparing the two is a lot like comparing apples and
oranges. My point? It's not an accurate comparison!

MYTH: Nurses just take orders.
Truth: In many cases, nurses function in a major
role in healthcare, as doctors do. Nurses are responsible
in managing the care of patients, which for example,
involves reviewing a patient's chart for important

information like lab values and other test results. Yet a nurse does not affirm a formal diagnosis; medical diagnoses are confirmed by the doctor. But nurses perform many clinical tasks such as providing care for their patients. Doctors do not spend a lot of time on taking a patient's blood pressure, or drawing blood for testing, but nurses do. Nurses perform ongoing assessments of patients and while hospitalized, patients have ongoing monitoring from a nurse. Part of monitoring involves carrying out the physician's written orders.

MYTH: Nursing school is for women only.

Truth: Although the industry has historically been mostly female dominated, data suggests that men are in the nursing profession, and it is not all dominated by women, as some would believe. According to a recent article published by Ameritech College of Healthcare, the notion that all nurses are women is still a very common misconception among most people employed in fields outside of healthcare, and it's simply not true, especially in today's contemporary workforce. The American Association of Colleges of Nursing states that men represent 6.6% of the U.S. nursing workforce, with men making up 11.4% of baccalaureate and 9.9% of master's nursing programs. In doctoral programs, 6.8% of students in research-focused programs and 9.4% of students in practice-focused programs are men.

MYTH: There is simply no room to grow in nursing. I'll be stuck doing the same job forever — taking care of patients at the bedside.

Truth: Ameritech College of Healthcare has published that there are currently more than 100 specialties in nursing and there are numerous advanced degree options; therefore, nurses are allotted the flexibility to change their career path as often as they want. Many nurses start clinically, at the bedside, develop their experience in a particular specialized area (I suggest medical-surgical area) and then pursue working in a specialty area. You'll find after you read through the contents of this book that there are various areas of specialization that a nurse can choose. There is absolutely no such thing as a dead-end career path for nurses. There is always plenty of room for growth, but be warned that growing in the nursing field always requires higher education and many years of hands-on training and experience. Later in this book, we will discuss what other career options you can pivot toward after gaining some experience in the field and perhaps an advanced degree or two.

MYTH: I will not be able to find a job after graduation.

Truth: Many new grads find it a challenge in landing their first nursing job after graduation and licensure. This myth is only partially true because employers are hiring those with experience, which a new grad does not have. There is a workaround to this. I recommend while you are in nursing school to take on a part-time role at a hospital, clinic, or any healthcare facility such as a nursing home. By taking up the role as a student nurse assistant, a nurses' aide, a hospital transport, or a pharmacy tech in a hospital, you gain experience — all while being in a healthcare environment. Employers look at this as positive experience.

•

The goal of the guide is to assist the individual in preparing for the process of studying nursing and to also, perhaps, help one in recognizing the need for adjustments to their lives when studying for the rigorous academic and clinical work that can and does affect even the best and brightest nursing students today. I truly believe nursing isn't for everybody, particularly those who do not give much thought to whether they can do this. One point I want to emphasize is that there is no *right* or *wrong* decision when it comes to choosing the profession or not choosing the profession. There are, however, right and wrong reasons for choosing to attend nursing school, which will be covered in the following chapters. This book is not meant as a persuasive argument for entering or not entering nursing school. It is merely a handbook for helping someone decide whether it is right for them or not. So do your homework and prepare yourself for a rewarding journey in nursing school.

Many do not know what nursing is all about, and time after time, I find quite a few individuals entering into the profession at a loss. Somewhere during their quest to attend nursing school, nobody ever told them what nursing was really about, what being a nurse entailed, or that they may have to roll up their sleeves and get their hands a little bit dirty from time to time — and I do mean dirty.

Nursing curricula include a theory and clinical part of a nursing program. The theory portion of the program is the classroom part where students study the history and theory of nursing and the clinical part (what I teach) of the curriculum is where one will introduce their nursing skills in a hospital, clinic, and other healthcare environments.

Additionally, today more and more nursing schools are including simulation portions of study as part of their program by developing simulation centers onto their nursing school campuses. This is a good thing, as it allows for more hands-on training for the student.

Simulation centers utilize high fidelity manikins operated by simulation technicians. A simulation manikin functions as a live patient, giving students an illusion that the mechanical device is real and as close to real life as a prop possibly can get. Simulation centers are set-up and arranged as hospital room settings to be as realistic as possible. Students are offered the opportunity to practice and develop their nursing skills prior to attending their clinical settings, which has proven to be very helpful in their training. So, my recommendation is for you to apply to schools that have simulation centers at part of the curricula.

I have seen time after time where students are faced with starting off in a nursing program and have absolutely no idea what to expect from it. This guide will aid the student or the new nurse through the experience of deciding whether the decision to become a nurse is the right one for him or her.

One of the most important questions to ask yourself is, "What makes me want to enroll in nursing school? Why do I want to become a nurse?" There are many reasons that students choose nursing as a career path, and no not all of them were created equally. Unfortunately, there are some students who choose to enroll with the high hopes of meeting and marrying the fictitious "Dr. McDreamy," which is something some students aspire to far too often to simply ignore. Others enroll simply because they want to "make a lot of money." Each time I hear this, I cannot help but smile and chuckle under my breath when a student remarks in that way. While nursing can certainly be a lucrative profession, no successful soon-to-be-nurse will have a meaningful and satisfying career if their primary motive is money.

Because of these reasons, I have been overcome by a compelling motivation of mine for writing this book to reform the nursing industry and return to what the profession was years ago when I first entered it. When I began my career, nursing was much, much different from what it is today. The healthcare industry and clinicians placed the highest value on caring for patients with very good outcomes. Unfortunately, times have changed. In today's, society, I'm seeing more and more clinicians lacking the compassion and care-driven behaviors to provide excellent care for patients. Needless to say, this can be problematic for everyone involved in the long run, and healthcare is currently facing the hard line reality. The shortage of nurses and shortage of nurse faculty does equal to care delivered.

In conducting my research for this book, many of my students gave a distinct reason to why they decide to enroll in nursing school. Some students enroll because, at some point in their lives, they have had the unfortunate experience of losing a loved one, thus the sheer reminiscence of that person's existence gives them the strong temptation to give back to the community in some way. Typically, those aforementioned students have witnessed their ill loved ones being cared for by nurses and during which times have thought to themselves, "I can do that," or "I want to do that." These individuals are still overwhelmed with emotions and grief of their loss and want to contribute back. While their reason for wanting to do this work is understandable, it may not always be the best reason for choose nursing as a career.

Although nursing is very hard work, the truth of the matter is that you can do anything you set your mind to, and the primary goal of this book is to assist you along the path.

In being on this writing journey, I did not realize until recently that I began to feel compelled to write a manuscript because of the mere fact that I was becoming more and more despondent of the vast population of students enrolling in the many nursing programs. Today's enrollees are entering into the profession with a variety of academic backgrounds but with little to no exposure clinically in healthcare. Some students have remarked to me they had never stepped foot in a hospital, so you can imagine the cultural shock on the first day of their clinical course.

As an adjunct professor, I've successfully taught hundreds of nursing students over the years, and I have personally seen students enroll in my clinical course not having basic nursing skills, skills required in the delivery of basic nursing care like offering a patient a urinal, assisting a patient onto a bedpan, or performing oral or morning care to a patient.

On the first day of their clinical rotation I have seen many students struggle. Why, you ask? Because they did not know a major part of nursing would require touching a patient. To even my surprise, I could not understand why they did not know this very important information, because a great part of nursing is assessing your patients, which means you will have to lay hands on that individual. Hello!

Let's face it folks; part of being a nurse and practicing in the role does require one to "Touch" and handle another human being, a stranger, someone with whom you are not familiar, like a ... "Patient." Also, nursing involves a willingness to SERVE and to CARE! Provide your care to a stranger. You have now entered into a career as a caregiver (please look up the definition of this term, study it, and familiarize yourself with it well).

So, do you have what it takes to enter the highly

competitive and demanding field of nursing? This book will guide you through the process and help you decide if it is right for you. At the end of this book, you will know whether you're making the right decision to enter the field. That is my goal and promise to you, but to start, I must begin with a bit of information from a former student of mine, Jennifer R., who is a recent graduate and successful BSN, RN. In this statement, Jennifer clearly states what it takes to be successful and to really thrive in such a competitive field filled with obstacles.

Jennifer states: *"I believe the three most important skills to have to be successful in nursing school are hard work, organization, and open mindedness. Nursing school was very challenging; unlike anything I have done before. I would have never been successful without putting in many hours of studying and keeping on task. Having an open mind is critical due to the different healthcare employees, nurses, preceptors, and teachers you'll meet with different techniques and teaching styles."*
Jennifer R., BSN, RN, 2014 graduate

After reading Jennifer's words, do you feel you have what it takes? Are you ready for the challenge? Are you prepared to look inside yourself and find out if this is the right move for you? Are you prepared to put away all the myths and stereotypes you may have heard about nursing and finally find out what nursing school and being an actual registered nurse is really like? If you answered "yes" to these questions then you are on the right track and ready for what is to come.

CHAPTER 1

So you wanna be a nurse, eh?

One of the primary goals of this book is to help potential nursing students decide whether nursing is the right field for them or not; therefore, the main question you need to ask yourself is if nursing is right for you. Some students immediately say "yes," while others seem unsure. It might be easy for you to say "yes," but in my experience, I have encountered many students enrolling in nursing schools who are too often unaware of what nursing is actually about, or what the profession even entails. This is partially due to the media and to certain pop culture television shows casting the profession in a light that is mostly fictitious and often gives an inaccurate portrayal of the profession, as Hollywood tends to do. This notion is highly problematic for a plethora of reasons. The last thing the nursing profession needs is more and more people choosing to enroll in nursing school with a false sense of reality as to what the profession actually entails, which is precisely what is happening today in our culture.

Additionally, this book was also written for anyone who is contemplating the decision to enroll in nursing school, whether it is someone fresh out of high school or college, or is a seasoned professional who has decided to give up a lucrative career from another field and looking to make a switch into the healthcare industry. After reading this book, the reader will have had a no-nonsense look into studying in the field of nursing, and have made the decision of whether nursing is a career for them. I believe you must first have a profound sense of drive, motivation, and passion to be successful in any credible nursing program. I say this because nursing is one of the most serious professions you could ever work in.

I have a unique perspective of nursing primarily from

my knowledge of teaching clinical nursing. I have strong beliefs regarding my role and the students who take my class. Throughout the term I aim to give students the ins-and-outs of nursing with a no-nonsense approach. Guiding students on a clinical site and providing instruction for them in an effort to develop their clinical skills is something I would not trade for anything. What helps is for students to come to clinical with a positive mind for a good experience and importantly, come to learn the real nursing. This guide is a depiction of what's real about nursing. Do you want to be a nurse to help people, or are your motives shifting toward the money or the dream of marrying a handsome doctor? After all, being a nurse means that your primary job duties revolve around interacting with sick people! There are so many amazing things I have experienced from my time as a nurse. It is a great profession, yet it may not be for everyone. Let's first take a look at what types of people decide to enroll in nursing school.

WHO DECIDES TO ENROLL IN NURSING SCHOOL?

So, who decides to enroll in nursing school, anyway? Good question! After reading about the influx of people enrolling in nursing school with a false sense of reality, many of you are probably wondering what kind of person decides to enroll in nursing school to begin with.

First and foremost, nursing is not a "job." Nursing is a profession, a career, a life decision, and a full-time life commitment, to say the least. It is unlike any other career and it is something that an outsider (or anyone who is not a nurse) will never truly understand. If you are a nurse and you talk to non-nurse friends or family members of yours, they will never truly be able to understand what it is that you do, or how difficult your job truly is and what it entails. Ask yourself, what is my perception of nursing? Do I know the history behind nursing? Am I truly passionate about helping people, working long hours, and providing quality care to the patients in my care?" These questions are quite critical when determining if entering the nursing profession is the right move for you. I must say in my younger years, I watched a lot of television — primarily drama programming from the 70's, which involved medical emergencies shows like "M.A.S.H", "Emergency," and "St. Elsewhere" starring a young Denzel Washington. During this time, there I was, intensely watching weekly where I engulfed myself in every episode following Denzel Washington's character as a doctor in training in a fictional hospital setting known as St. Eligius. I knew from that moment that a career in healthcare was a career path I wanted to be on. (There I said it: I watched too much Television!) Such programs like those today are edited for your entertainment, so please do not base your decision to attend nursing school around a TV show.

Because as I have stated, nursing is certainly not just a career to me. It is my life, my passion, and profession, which I take extremely seriously, and so should anyone who is even considering becoming a nurse. Nurses work in an environment that is surrounded by serving others and taking care of their needs; you're responsible for those individuals in your care. It is no surprise that caring for patients is serious business, as being a nurse involves playing a substantial role in the patient's care and overall prognosis of their ailment(s).

While most people believe that doctors are the heroes in a hospital setting, nurses are the backbone of any functioning, successful healthcare structure. As a nurse, I carry intensity, drive, and passion into my daily role as a clinical nurse and instructor. I am recognized as a strict, no-nonsense clinician and educator where those whom I precept often remark on how much they have learned. I absolutely love teaching students who are passionate and eager about learning all there is about nursing care specifically. Nursing can be a complex profession; however nursing is what you and only you put into the profession.

Each new term, I always begin my class at the commencement of each semester to make a point to ask my students the question of why they have decided to enroll in nursing school. Their responses give me the background information related to their perception of nursing, and what they hope to gain from a career in nursing. From this information I know what to expect as their clinical instructor. For the students, their answers to my initial question are usually always driven by passion, most notably the students who decided to become nurses because they had a nurse in their life that played an integral role in their family member's care. During one class session, a student informed me that she decided to become a nurse because her mother had cancer two years prior and it was a dedicated nurse who stood by her bedside each day, providing care. It was clear that she was very compassionate, and I had a strong feeling that her drive and compassion toward sick individuals would be enough to carry her through the rather difficult times that the profession called for. Anytime I ask students that question, my hope is that they are pursuing the profession to provide excellent, safe patient care.

WHY DECIDE TO ENROLL?

I imagine you are currently reading this book because you are wondering whether you should enroll in nursing school. Maybe you are quite sure of the decision, maybe you're on the fence and looking for that one special reason to attend, or maybe you have just enrolled. Whatever the case, those who decide to enroll in nursing school do so for a variety of reasons.

Myia T., a nurse of five years states: *"I enjoy helping people and learning about the disease and illnesses. Also, I enjoy the close interaction with people on a day-to-day basis. When I saw the lack of interaction doctors had with patients, I knew I would rather be a nurse."*
Myia T. RN, 2011 graduate

This information is critical, as I have tried to explain that doctors, often times, have very little communication time with their patients. A newly graduated nurse should have a mission to provide excellent, quality care to his/her patients. This care is delivered by interacting closely with patients. The doctor may enter the room and offer their patient information about their diagnoses, answer questions about their plan of care, and leave the room. Yet it is the nurse who really develops a bond with the patient because patients are in their care throughout their shift and sometime for days. Because doctors spend such a limited time with patients, this makes it difficult to build a strong physician-patient relationship. But nurses are more accessible, and most people would agree patients feel more comfortable asking the nurse to explain something that they didn't understand from the doctor mostly because of a feeling of uneasy intimidation. Because of this, there is trust established between the nurse and the patient, which builds a relationship and respect.

"A strong, perhaps overwhelming desire to quickly run to the aid of a patient who needs treating or care is one of the most important factors for my choosing to become a nurse".
Edyta C., a 2014 graduate from nursing school and current clinician, describes her motivation as just that.

She states: *"I enrolled in nursing school due to the fact that I have a strong desire to help people and it is my path in life. I wanted to be a nurse because I enjoy being around people in their times of need, and I get internal satisfaction by serving those that need help. I remember when I did some volunteer work for a hospital, I realized my passion for nursing. I believe that the cure for many of the people's illnesses is not just in medicine, it is in the care that they receive as patients in hospitals and their homes. This is where I believe that I can make a great difference in people's lives by helping them recover from their ailments."*

This statement makes it quite clear that Edyta has chosen the nursing profession for the right reasons, and her attitude and desire to help others is reflected in her work each day. Furthermore, she describes her motivation as being fueled by the passion and love for people and internal satisfaction by serving those in need. That, my friend, is a recipe for success in my book!

There is also a plethora of individuals who graduate from a four-year institution and have entered the working world in other fields, only to find themselves stuck in dead-end jobs and wanting more of a sense of satisfaction within their careers. This is quite common, and can work to your advantage because there are quite a few nursing tracks of curricula and for this group of individuals there is the ABSN, Accelerated Baccalaureate of Science in Nursing track, which we will discuss later in the chapter covering the variety of nursing programs. In my perception, many nurses who enter the field later in life or after having completed an undergraduate degree from another field are focused and bring to nursing life experiences.

A former student Megan M., RN and 2015 ABSN graduate makes a compelling argument when she states: *"I enrolled in nursing school because when I graduated in 2012 with my other Bachelor degree, I remember sitting at graduation and feeling very unsatisfied with my decision. I had been pre-nursing major and changed majors the end of my sophomore year and it resulted in a lot of disappointment in myself and regret, so I made changes to get into a nursing program. My primary motivation was that I was still young and I didn't want to live my entire life thinking 'what if I went to nursing school,' so instead I acted on it."*
Megan M. RN, 2015 ABSN graduate

In this instance, Megan made the decision to pursue a four-year degree in another field, yet quickly knew upon graduating that nursing school was the right decision for her. Luckily, for Megan, she didn't waste any more time before enrolling. She knew what she wanted to do and she made a strong effort to make that dream a reality. While each and every person has their own personal motivation for choosing to enroll in nursing school, there are always those individuals who look at nursing as a calling.

Registered nurse, Modestine, says it best when she states: *"My primary motivation was my personal view of the nursing as a sacred profession. Every day, they touched the lives of so many people in a very unique way. In the nurse role, sometimes, we bring a ray of light into lives that have been shadowed by the burden of diseases and discomfort. I enrolled in nursing school because I enjoy taking care of the vulnerable population, the elderly and the underserved."*
Modestine, N., RN, 2015 BSN graduate

This is the kind of attitude that almost always guarantees that a nurse will be successful in their career, most notably because the nurse has clearly shown that they are willing to put the patient's needs far above their own. This is the building block for what makes a great nurse, and that is something that every nurse should take very seriously. There needs to be more nurses with strong attitudes like Modestine's, as that is truly an asset for nursing as a career choice. Deanne B.'s story is somewhat similar to those who seek out nursing because of their distaste of the lack of passion they found while pursuing careers in other fields, which is more common than people think.

She states: *"Before enrolling in nursing school I was working in behavioral healthcare, but I was bored and felt like it was not something I was passionate about. I wanted to do something that I knew would complete me. I have always known I wanted to work in healthcare, but I was not sure what field I wanted to go into. I have many nurses in my family and I also had a personal health experience that made me want to go into nursing to help others."*
Deanne B., RN, BSN, 2015 graduate

While just about every nurse I've ever spoken with has their own personal reasons for choosing to enroll in nursing school, there are those individuals who find their interest for nursing while volunteering, which for some, is the first time they've had the honor of caring for someone in the sense that a nurse cares for their patients. Lisa B., a 2015 graduate, cites volunteering at a hospital as the catalyst for making her realize that a career in the nursing field was the right decision for her.

Lisa states: *"I volunteered at a local hospital for 40 hours in high school and knew I wanted to be a nurse after volunteering on every nursing unit. I fell in love with nursing very young. I already had a passion since I volunteered and knew that was what I wanted to do for the rest of my life. I loved medicine and knew nursing was for me."*
Lisa B., RN, 2015 graduate

The main common denominator for these three individuals is prior to becoming a nurse they each were employed and gained some experience in working in a healthcare environment. This is key, because it also aided in their decisions in choosing nursing as a career. So, have you ever volunteered? I would recommend this noble experience. You can always follow in Lisa's footsteps and volunteer at a local hospital. While you will not get to do everything that a nurse will (for obvious reasons), you will gain some exposure into what it's like to work in a hospital around patients who need care, which is experience that can prove to be invaluable.

WHY ENROLL? WHY IS BEING A NURSE A GOOD IDEA?

Why should you enroll in nursing school, anyway? Great question! Most of the times when students approach me about this topic, they already know that they want to be a nurse; however, they need to also know that there are ample job opportunities that they will have upon finishing their degree and entering the nursing field. The truth is that there are so many opportunities for today's new graduates in nursing.

Listed below are only some of the vast numbers of reasons that it's a good idea to enroll in nursing school:

1) Opportunity: According to a 2015 data study performed by the Bureau of Labor Statistics, nursing is single handedly the fastest-growing occupation in the United States. In fact, nurses make up the majority of the healthcare industry. That number is 3.1 million and growing. The projected employment growth for nurses over the next decade is 20.1 percent, leaving over 581,000 more nursing jobs by the year 2018. This is excellent news for new nurses, and those considering nursing as a career. Registered Nurses meet America's healthcare needs on every level because there are many opportunities for job prospects. This accounts for a 22% increase in expected nursing jobs from 2008 to 2018, which is far higher than many other booming industries. One of the primary reasons to explain this increase in demand is the fact that the nursing population is aging and there is a shrinking workforce. Those of you reading this book now in 2016 could presumably enroll in nursing school and be finished by that time, making you right on the cusp of the job boom.

2) Options: One of the many excellent benefits to becoming a nurse is the vast array of flexible work options

that you have available. Nursing allows you a variety of different choices such as where to work, which advanced degree(s) to obtain, or specific areas of specialty that you can become certified in; a certification offers you as a nurse additional options and perks when it comes to marketing yourself. There are countless nursing areas to specialize in, and there is almost always a shortage of these specialties, so if you have a specialty, you will be extremely employable and will have the flexibility to work in almost any field of nursing that you choose. In times of nursing shortages, which is usually the case as long as I can remember, today's nurses are armed with more hiring power that can afford them generous earning potential and hiring perks.

3) Work environment: As a nurse, you will have many options as to where you choose to work. Hospitals like academic facilities are very good environments to work for a new nurse. Here you can gain a great deal of knowledge building, as well as see and provide care for patients who have anything from textbook to rare illnesses and diseases. These are great learning opportunities. Some nurses choose to work in clinics and doctor's offices, outpatient facilities, and for home-health services. I see this in senior nurses, nurses who have been there, who as they say, have done their time and are looking for areas of work where the environment is calmer and the work load tends to be not so strenuous. When you begin your nursing career, you will have the option to work in any of the aforementioned environments, and you will have the freedom to survey each of the environments to find one that is a perfect fit for you.

4) Flexible Career: Currently there are more than a hundred nursing specialties and a substantial number of advanced nursing degrees available to obtain; therefore, there are many nurses who often pivot to

new specialties within different scopes of medicine after beginning their career such as, Medical-Surgical nursing, which comprises 80% of the nursing workforce and is an area that I recommend for a new nurse to start his/her career. From here, after working in an area for a substantial period of time, a nurse can figure out what areas appeal the most. Nurses tend to move to other specialty areas after earning advanced degrees, in an effort to continue advancing their career options. By furthering their education and training into a specialized field of interest, a nurse can continue to create his/her earning power because, as mentioned earlier, the more marketable the nurse becomes, the more career options there will be available.

5) Flexible Schedule: Okay, so here's the deal: nurses work long hours! While most of us already know that, we also need to acknowledge that there's usually a good deal of flexibility in a nurse's schedule. Although nurses tend to work long hours, they also tend to have flexible schedules as well. The sporadic schedule of a nurse will really depend on what specialty area or what work facility you choose; usually beginning nurses tend to choose shifts of 10 and 12 hours, which can offer you additional work days off during the week.

Nurses can typically work three 12-hour or four 10-hour shifts per week and that's on one job location (Lol!). I say this because I've seen nurses take on additional shifts at other facilities for extra income. However, to those who want to work a "normal" work week there are five 8-hour work days per week offered as well. Nurses with families tend to occupy this form of schedule. Having the freedom of a flexible schedule is a huge perk of being a nurse, and oftentimes will lead to an increase in employee morale and overall career satisfaction. In addition, flexible schedules are highly advantageous to working parents who have to work during specific hours in order to attend to their childcare or family needs. For example, many nurses choose the 12-hour shift work days because the three work days a week can free up their long commute to work, or their options to work weekdays, weekends, or a hybrid of both is a better work schedule for their lives at the time.

6) Flexible Location: Flexible location, anyone? Yes, please! The healthcare industry is in very high demand all across the globe, and there is a vast shortage of nurses in almost every geographical area. Essentially, this means that after you receive your degree, you will be free to work in any city, state, or even country you choose (after you apply for and receive a license). Ever heard of a travel nurse? Some nurses choose the option as a travel nurse (some travel agencies require at least a year of experience). This option offers nurses great perks, like housing stipends and supplemental pay at higher rates, to name a couple. There is a need for nurses everywhere, and this is an option that you can certainly use to your advantage.

CHANGES IN THE NURSING PROFESSION

Every industry morphs, transitions, and changes over a given amount of time and nursing is no different. One of the greatest changes within the nursing world is the introduction of technology. When I started nursing 20 years ago, paper documentation was the standard form of documenting a patient's care. Nurses during that time were subjected to deciphering orders written by doctors that were very poorly written to the point where you and your coworkers would huddle to interpret, sometimes taking bets on what the order for the patient was. Since the revolution of computer documentation, I have to say I couldn't be happier! Computer documentation has proven to have made nursing and healthcare much more efficient and effective for those in the field. There is a cornucopia of new devices that are being introduced and integrated into healthcare facilities, which have the ability to enhance a patient's experience, like kiosk patient check-ins for procedures, and also iPad use for check–ins for doctor's office appointments or same day procedure check-ins. Many hospitals and doctor's offices are beginning to provide this technology and find it is highly effective for the flow of their practice. Patients will find their information remains secure and confidential.

If you're reading this book now and you have not yet attended nursing school, there is a high probability that by the time you are ready to search for employment as a nurse, there will be many more changes than what are listed above. Technology is making one of time's oldest professions even more exciting. Fear not nurse wannabe, technology is not to replace the human or the compassionate factor of nursing. That means please do not treat the computer as a patient and I say this because in my experience I see the Millennial and Gen Xers doing this a lot, they gravitate to the COMPUTER! You cannot assess the computer folks, please assess the patient and not the computer, more on this later. I foresee nursing will continue to require the hands-on, skilled individuals to do the job for some time.

CHAPTER 2

Other reasons for attending nursing school

As you are probably aware, not all decisions for going to nursing school are created equal. There are good decisions and bad decisions, and the purpose of this chapter is to help you decide whether your reasons for choosing to attend nursing school are good reasons or not-so-good reasons. The sole purpose of designing this chapter was for you to stop and think about the real reason you want to attend nursing school; therefore, please evaluate yourself honestly and critically. While I have heard all of these reasons during my tenure, it's important to note what makes these good and bad decisions and why they are important. Below is a list of various good and bad reasons that I have heard over the years and why they are considered "good" or "bad" reasons for choosing this field and yes, I have really heard all of these reasons from various students over the years!

GOOD REASONS TO ATTEND NURSING SCHOOL

You Want To Do Nursing: Ask yourself, "How long have I been contemplating the decision to enroll in nursing school?" Sometimes I will speak with students or just potential students and some of them have had the dream in their hearts to go into nursing since they were old enough to know what a nurse does. Others find themselves with the dream in their hearts later in life, most oftentimes after they have already completed a degree in another discipline and haven't found the level of job satisfaction that they were looking for. Also, some are still suffering the effects of the tough economy of several years ago. These individuals are often unhappy with their careers or loss of careers so they find the answer in a career in nursing.

You must want to do nursing, and most importantly you must want to be a nurse for you, not your friend, not your mother, not your grandmother, or simply ... not your culture. The dream must be yours, not anyone else's; otherwise, you'll be disappointed, even if you somehow make it through the rigorous, unforgiving curriculum that nursing school is known to offer.

You Have A Willingness to Serve Others: The keyword in the title is "others." Why? Simple! Nursing isn't about your willingness to serve yourself; it's about your willingness to serve your patients and to provide the best possible care for them that is within the standards of practice. At times when you're not working, friends, family, and your peers will call for medical advice. If ever a situation occurs when that nurse is around, they are often expected to use their medical training to take care of situations as they arise. When it comes to care, you will become the sole designated spokesperson for all of your family members. They will trust you to help them. Welcome their questions with an open mind and an open heart. True nurses love helping others, whether they are on the clock or off the clock.

You Have Compassion Toward Others: When was the last time you were listening to the news and you heard about someone dying from cancer, a tragic accident where someone lost their life, or simply had a family member stricken with an illness that seemed almost hopeless? Did you quickly think about something else, or did you stop and wonder about how you could help? Did you move forward with your day, or did you picture yourself on the scene providing optimum care and comfort to someone that needed it? One of the most important things a nurse can possibly have is compassion toward others, toward strangers or a loved one. Recently I watched a commencement address titled "Maintain Humility" presented by Dr. Jennifer Arnold in 2014 at West Coast University, a school that comprises of future healthcare professionals. Dr. Arnold is a little person with skeletal dysplasia, a bone disease, who has endured and overcame more than 30 orthopedic surgeries to correct her condition. She spoke clearly to the graduating class and challenged each of them to "Remember why you are in the field."

In her speech Dr. Arnold urged graduates to offer their patients humility and compassion and when caring for patients to use their talents to collaborate as a team. Maintain courage to be humble and true to yourself and your patients. Approach healthcare with pride, joy, and humility. You can make a difference in the lives of your patients with constant self-awareness. Know your limitations, have openness and empathy, and maintain gratitude for the privilege to serve. The ability to understand and feel another person's pain is openness. It is okay to show empathy for your patients; this is not a sign of weakness. Last, keep in mind to treat your patients as you would want to be treated or how you would want a family member or friend to be treated when receiving care and not to demonstrate entitlement. This was a wonderful message to the graduating class and I believe a true testament to the spirit of nursing. Healthcare — specifically nursing — will give back what you bring to it and if you choose to bring those above qualities to the profession then nursing will reward you also.

You Are Ready For the Challenges of Nursing: One of the best predispositions for success in nursing school is being ready for a challenge, because that is exactly what nursing school is going to be. Some ambitious students I've come across throughout the years thrive on being involved in challenges, and others not so much. As I've stated before, nursing is very challenging, and if you have not learned that yet, you soon will. The most successful nursing students and nurses I've had the pleasure of working with are those who see a challenge as a learning opportunity and yes, as nurses you can still learn a thing or two. As I was saying, in nursing, each and every day is vastly different from the day before, ensuring that those who are up for a challenge will find that the nursing career is a perfect fit for one's curiosity coupled with the desire to help others, and be a team player.

Passion: Passion is both an interesting and unique phenomenon. While most of us believe that we have passion, only few of us actually do. Nursing is a career that is utterly built upon the notion of having a strong, compelling sense of passion. While you may be able to pass the required classes and exams, if you lack passion for helping and watching others heal as a direct result of the excellent care that you provide them, then you're probably going to have some challenges as a nurse.

BAD REASONS TO ATTEND NURSING SCHOOL

So we've just spent some time discussing some of the good reasons to attend nursing school, but it just wouldn't be right if we didn't do the same for the bad reasons. The purpose of this section is to make sure you're entering the field for the right reasons; not the wrong ones.

Money: I would have to say money does have a part in one's decision in enrolling in a nursing program but the heart and soul of nursing is about care delivered. If dollar signs cloud your vision when the thought of becoming a nurse crosses your mind, then this could be an issue. Later in this book, we will discuss the current statistics of nursing salaries and yes, the salary is quite generous, especially if you choose to advance your education and specialize. That being said, you're in for a rude awakening if you're only getting into nursing for monetary reasons. This is a common mistake that I hear far too often from students to ignore, and it is one that I detest and highly advocate against. Please do not go into the nursing field solely for the money because you could soon find the work harder than you perceived, and the otherwise "fat" paychecks will not seem like a lot for all of the hard work that you're putting in. Although the salary for a nurse can be quite generous, and nurses can certainly earn a good paycheck, it is important to know that no successful nurse is only in it for the money.

Respect: While it's certainly true that nurses are highly respected in the medical field and by most people in general, simply attending nursing school with the high hopes that someone will respect you is a plan that is seemingly doomed for failure. Remember nursing is about the patient.

It's The Only Stable Career Option: It's rare that a student enrolls because it's their only option, but I've certainly heard it before. Very few times in life is there only one option, and nursing is no different. There are many, many career choices for someone to choose from. Please do not attend nursing school because you believe it's your only option. Even if you somehow finish your degree and land a job, you will not be happy with your career and it will take a negative toll on the rest of your life — which will only lead to a life of perpetual unhappiness. So be wise about your decision.

You Couldn't Get Into Medical School: Did you apply to medical school but didn't get in? If this is your situation, just know that being a doctor is not the same as being a nurse, as being a nurse requires much more hands-on care with patients because nurses spend more time with patients than doctors. You will know right from the beginning if nursing is a fit for you. Let's face it, nurses have a prominent role in a patient's healing and their care is needed. Case in point: Nurses are a great reference source because of their strong sense of clinical judgment. They are often asked their opinions and recommendations from resident physicians (if you work in an academic facility), nursing colleagues, and others this is multidisciplinary care for patients. If you want to know something then ask a nurse! Sorry, doctor.

Your Parents/Family Members Think You Should Go: I'm finding many of my students current and past — made the decision to enroll in a nursing program because of the advice of a parent, other family member, a friend, and now more and more there is a cultural influence in a person's career choice for nursing. Make sure you weigh all of the pros and cons when making your decision.

Your Favorite TV Character Is a Nurse and It Looks and Sounds "Cool": Hollywood has a great way of altering the perception of reality. They do it in movies, books, radio, the media, and television all the time. There are many popular medical-based dramas where the nursing profession is depicted. You know them, Grey's Anatomy, Nurse Jackie, and in my day it was, St. Elsewhere, starring the handsome young Denzel Washington. Yep, but unfortunately, that aforementioned depiction is only a facade for the lens of the camera, and for your entertainment purposes, of course. It is not real, and you should not be persuaded to enter the field based on what you saw last night on House, a TV character doctor who tackles health mysteries. It's interesting when students enroll in nursing school because of a Hollywood movie or television show that has shaped their perception of the field. Such students do not have a clear perception of what nursing really entails.

So, forget everything you've ever seen in movies or television about nursing. It's not the same! It's not reality!

Your Best Friend Is Going To Nursing School; Therefore, You Should Too!: Believe it or not, I've heard this reason before, as well. Just like the other "bad" reasons in this list, this reason is simply no exception. While I understand that a person might want to enter the same career path as a friend, nursing is not meant for everyone. No career field in the world is. Please make sure the decision is yours and yours alone and you are choosing it because it is right for you.

•

Do any of these reasons sound familiar? Hopefully, your reason or reasons for attending nursing school are in the list of "good" reasons. If you choose to go into nursing for the right reasons, there is little doubt that you will have a fulfilling career. If you do, however, find your reasons for thinking about enrolling in nursing school to be one or more of those on the "bad" list, then you probably should reconsider your decision.

CHAPTER 3

Nursing involves what, exactly?

Since many of the students who enroll in nursing school are unaware of the rigorous academic demands of the coursework in addition to what being a nurse actually entails, this chapter will assist you in getting an accurate depiction of what being a nurse involves. Nursing involves touching another human being, not just physically, but mentally and emotionally as well. There have been several times in my career when a patient has shown their gratitude for the care I've provided and because of this, I know that I had a substantial impact on their recovery and healing. While there are some people who may possess technical or medical knowledge it takes to become a nurse, you also have to be able to have strong bedside manner to successfully serve your patient's needs. Here is where customer service comes into play. Additionally, a huge part of nursing involves assessing your patients physically. If you have a problem in physically touching a stranger, then I am sorry to say that nursing just may not be the right profession for you.

Over the years that I have successfully managed other nurses, occasionally there were a few nurses who were very knowledgeable and book smart individuals, yet they lacked something that is critical for being successful as a nurse: assessment, which involves thinking critically. By critical thinking, a nurse must be able to respond, to react to a patient's changing condition, which requires critical thinking skills coupled with assessment skills. This is nursing in a nutshell.

Nursing also involves showing compassion toward total strangers. Think of it like this: You're a nurse who has a patient in your care who requires assistance with feeding, giving them a bath, administering their medication, offering a bedpan, cleaning up after them, and the list continues. Some nurses are quite comfortable with this and enjoy the feeling of taking care of someone in this way, however others may not be comfortable with such tasks; well folks, this is nursing.

It is important to mention an all too often observation: Many nursing students are quite timid afraid, and frankly, uncomfortable touching and providing care to complete strangers. I mentioned this earlier in the book, but want to explore it in this section. When I asked some of them why, they simply stated that they had no problem taking care of their friends or family members when they were needed, but when it was a stranger, they simply didn't feel right about it. They tell me, "I don't want to hurt or harm the person" ... their confidence is lacking and as student nurses I would like for you to know that being uncomfortable is something you can and will overcome if you work hard to overcome it. Yes, you can successfully provide care to total strangers, as it's unlikely that the hospital you work at is going to be filled with your friends and family. I can tell you right now that it won't be. The notion of hurting someone or harming an individual will be avoided if you practice safe, competent nursing care.

Prioritizing Care: Something you will learn early in your nursing career is how to manage and prioritize the care of your patients. This information is key and paramount to your skill base. I say this because perfecting this skill of prioritization has played a huge role in nursing, which I have become an advocate of. I'm often asked by students what areas of nursing would I recommend for a new graduate? My answer is Medical-Surgical nursing. Why medical-surgical nursing? Because of the nurse to patient staffing ratio, I believe the medical-surgical nursing units would afford a new nurse opportunities to develop and perfect those all too important skills of properly managing the care of their patients.

KEY COMPONENTS OF THE NURSING PROCESS

Some of the critical components of the nursing process include assessment, planning, implementation, and evaluation of care for patients. These are the hallmarks of nursing, and a successful nurse must be able to effectively acquire and manage each core fundamental component of the nursing process.

ASSESSING: Nursing assessment is a very important part of the holistic process of caring for a patient. During this time, the nurse gathers a substantial amount of information about their patient's physiological, psychological, biological, sociological, and emotional status and with this information, plans their care for the day. The assessment is the first step in the nursing process. Talking with and listening to your patients is part of the assessment process. As a nurse you will have to spend time listening to your patient. This is where the nurse begins to gather data to assist in their patient's care in the most efficient manner. It is also during this time where you as the nurse begin to build rapport and trust with your patients.

A Note Regarding Assessment: The biggest mistake I find new nurses making is their lack of physically assessing their patient. That's a no, no in my book. You must physically assess your patients at all times while they are in your care!

Assessment of a patient by a nurse is crucial and is a great part of a nurse's responsibility when a patient is in your care. New nurses must understand that assessing a patient's condition is an ongoing process — and is a required task of nursing practice. Yes, it does take skills, but the more opportunities you have to assess a patient the better you will become at it.

Why am I so big on this topic? Well if you haven't noticed, this is a pet peeve of mine. This is serious. A patient's clinical status can change at any given moment, sometimes instantly and this can become a nurse's nightmare if a condition has changed and the nurse has not looked in on their patient and assessed them.

Despite this, time after time, I continue to find students (and new nurses) sitting at the computer and documenting assessments on their patients that were not done. New nurses are too focused on completing tasks (another mistake new nurses make), and overlook the true issues and conditions of their patients.

Rule of thumb: Typically once you have received a report on your patient, the important next step you must take immediately is to go to the room and begin your assessment on you patient. This bit of information will provide you a baseline status of your patient's condition and assist in your plan of care for your shift. So please don't make this mistake. Assess your patients and not the computer.

I would have to say that this is the one piece of advice that I can give to you that will truly make a difference in your career.

PLANNING: Planning and managing care for your patients while they are in your care during your shift is key! When I starting nursing some years ago, care plans were the standard in managing patient care. Like doctors, nurses are responsible for developing a nursing diagnosis for their patients and with this diagnosis a care plan is created.

IMPLEMENTING: Implementing care to a patient is also a crucial part in nursing. For example, administering medications to a patient is an implementation process with standard steps to follow in completing this task. Also, there are other implementing tasks like pain management, managing the care of catheters, and performing dressing changes. The list goes on and on.

EVALUATING: A nurse must evaluate the care or what task has been implemented for their patient; the task must be reassessed. Part of evaluating for the best outcome of the patient, the nurse must assess and evaluate the implemented care to see if adjustments must be made. For example, if you administer a medication to a patient to treat his/her pain, at some point you must reassess the patient to evaluate what affects the medication had on the patient.

TEACHING: Here also, I must add the skill of patient teaching. In nursing, patient education is huge! Nurses perform a lot of patient education, be it giving information about self-care when homebound, or providing teaching about medication after discharge from the hospital, or even caring for surgical wounds and dressing changes for the promotion of healing and better patient outcomes. For a nurse, patient teaching is one of the greatest responsibilities and skills you must constantly develop.

TOOLS OF THE TRADE: BASIC EQUIPMENT NEEDS

It's no surprise being a successful nurse requires having the proper equipment on hand daily. You'll thank yourself for being prepared for unforeseen situations that occur in nursing. Just like any workman's occupation, the same applies in nursing. You will need extra equipment to make your workday easier and having the necessary accessories will aid in that. In order for a nurse to be fully equipped at all times during their shift, a nurse should have the following equipment on him/her at all times. Below I've listed a few must have pieces of equipment that you should not be without:

STETHOSCOPE: Every nurse should have a good quality stethoscope to assist in his/her patient assessments (once again here's where you will have to "touch" a patient) and in doing so you must have this gold standard piece of equipment. For a nurse, a stethoscope is used to assess their patients by listening to lung, heart, and abdominal sounds (and others). Most people always associate a doctor using the stethoscope, but in nursing this accessory is an essential item to have in your daily work place. When purchasing a stethoscope, it's important to be sure the device has both a bell and diaphragm feature, as each feature has different functions.

PEN LIGHT: For a practicing nurse, a pen light is used for your neurological assessments and is a vital assessment tool. Take it from me; you shouldn't be without one.

SCISSORS: A good pair of nursing scissors will always come in handy in opening tamper resistant packaging of supplies and also for removing clothing items in critical situations (yes, this happens). Make sure they are sharp, and make sure to always carry them with you. Find a quality pair of metal scissors; they are much stronger and work far better than their plastic counterparts.

HEMASTAT: Nursing involves working with tubing, i.e. IV tubings and others ... This item is a must-have and a lifesaver for a nurse for unclamping, twisting, and screwing difficult tubing and clamps, which often is a part of a nurse's daily routine. This is where your plumbing skills come into play.

SHOES: A nurse should have a good pair of quality walking shoes. This is a must! Please spend time to shop for a quality pair of shoes to your liking. Your feet will appreciate you, as you will be on your feet for many, many hours and having a comfortable pair of shoes is essential. Find a pair of enclosed (back and front) shoes, and make sure that they're comfortable and that you can spend long hours in them comfortably.

DO YOU HAVE THE SKILLS? BASIC NURSING SKILLS

The purpose of this section is for you to determine whether you have the skills to be successful in nursing school. When gathering the necessary amount of research for this book, I spent a considerable amount of time researching and surveying current students, former students, and colleagues of mine to gather a large amount of diverse data to bring to the table. One of the most important questions that I could ask is, "What skills do you need to be a successful nurse?" If you were to ask nurses this question, their responses would be all over the board.

Some students perform excellent in the theoretical part of the nursing curriculum. Yet they succumb to the heavy amount of stress that nursing students usually experience around their clinical skill performance. Myia T. understands the importance of being patient, confident, and relying on an excellent family support system for when you're feeling some stress by the requirements of the job.

Myia states: *"Patience, flexibility, confidence, and a support system via friends and/or family. You also need determination and organization and also, knowing how to relax is important."*
Myia T., RN, 2011 graduate

Myia graduated from nursing school a few years ago, and has since become absolutely dedicated to her work. She understands one of the most important things of being a nurse, which is patience. Throughout my career, I have met impatient nurses, whose lack of patience left a gap between them and their patients. Their patients are not as satisfied with their quality of care when they feel that their nurse is being impatient with them. When speaking with a patient during their initial visit, be patient and listen! Ask the patient questions, and allow her or him to speak for as long as needed in order to provide you with all of the information that you need. When administering medicine to someone and it's taking longer than expected, be patient. Do not make a patient feel uncomfortable by what appears to be you rushing them, even though you have other patients to attend to. Trust me, I know you're busy, but please do not give the patient that impression.

What about discipline, you might ask? After all, doesn't discipline play a role in a nurse's success? You bet it does! Are you disciplined? Don't worry; we haven't forgotten what an important factor discipline can be. Having discipline when it's needed is one of the most important skills an aspiring nurse can possess, as it is discipline that urges us to study and to work as hard as possible to accomplish our goals.

"A few skills I believe you need are discipline, confidence, and a positive outlook."
Megan M., RN, 2015 graduate

Megan's analysis of how discipline plays a vital role in determining what kind of nurse you will become is crucial. If you are disciplined, you will work hard and stay focused, otherwise, you will not. It's that simple. Learn to be disciplined and diligent in your work, and do not lose focus of what you are trying to accomplish and always, have confidence! A nurse who doesn't exude confidence in performing their role will not be well-received by their patients. Today patients are very intelligent and savvy in choosing a hospital or facility for their care. Patients today are more involved and concerned about the care that they expect at healthcare facilities and you should know that those who are delivering care and treatments are on high alert. Not only do patients have great expectations, but so does your employer. Hospitals and other health facilities are expected by governing agencies to provide care that is safe and competent or penalties are posed, which affect all levels of service including nursing.

So, always demonstrate confidence in your care. This skill is just as imperative as having the right tools to do your job. Additionally, nursing is about working independently and being a critical thinker. In your care you can develop this skill during your clinical sessions.

Modestine, a 2015 graduate states: *"In nursing school, it is important to be self-directed, self-disciplined, and self- determined. Striving for excellence and compassionate care could also add more power to the fuel of becoming an excellent nurse."*
Modestine, RN, 2015 graduate

Modestine is quite right in her statement, as striving for excellence and maintaining compassionate care at all times is a vital factor to being an excellent nurse; and of course, how could we forget about having excellent time-management skills? With the rigorous and demanding course load of a full-time nursing student, possessing excellent time-management skills is critical. Think about it for a moment: You have classes you have to attend, clinical you must attend, and a lot of outside studying that you need to do in order to properly prepare for the challenging examinations that you will face during nursing school.

Deanna B., a recent graduate, emphasizes the importance of time management when she states: *"Time-management, patience, flexibility, and good study habits."*
Deanna B., RN, BSN, 2015 graduate

There you have it; good study habits are essential! You need to know how you learn best in order to successfully develop proper study habits, as everyone retains information differently.

In addition to the invaluable recommendations above, Lisa B., adds to the conversation by showcasing the importance of studying and practicing the NCLEX questions before taking an exam.

Lisa states: *"There are three very important things that I would recommend. First, find tutors for all classes that took the class already. It really helps for them to give you a heads up for the class. Second, practice doing NCLEX questions before taking an exam. Finally, when studying, mostly focus on nursing interventions and make note cards out of them."*
Lisa B., RN, 2015 graduate

This advice is quite important, as many students do not realize nursing school is ongoing. Well after graduation you must still continue to study until you sit for and pass NCLEX.

CHALLENGES OF BEING A NURSE ... ONLY IF YOU ALLOW THEM TO BE

There are many reasons why I love the nursing profession, but it is as equally important for me to explain some of the challenges that nurses face in an attempt to paint an accurate picture of what being a nurse is all about. I should mention that an entire stand-alone book could be written on this subject.

Imagine knowing the etiology, classification, dosage, side effects, contraindications, and compatibility for the different medications out today. A nurse is expected to know this information. But do not fret or have an immediate concern. Just like all there is to know in nursing when it comes to developing your knowledge base on medication administration, it comes with time and practice. There are also multitudes of resources on site that will aide in enhancing this skill while you're performing this daily task. Many hospitals have multiple pharmacy satellites on site, and also pharmacy references at your fingertips on the facility's intranet program, something I didn't have when I started in nursing; paper documentation was around during that time.

Another challenge of being a nurse is simply that of balancing the many demands. As a nurse, you must learn how to be completely engaged in your work, but also learn how to find down time where you can recharge. Doing this can help you be a more effective and successful nurse, and once again, it's all about prioritizing and managing your care.

CHAPTER 4

Prerequisites to entering the field & changes in the industry

Out of all the prerequisites a person can have before entering the nursing profession, I believe the most critical one of them all is having some previous work experience in a hospital environment prior to enrolling in nursing school. Earlier, we discussed that it's certainly feasible to receive experience through volunteering in a hospital in an effort to gain some entry-level exposure to the nursing field, which can be an excellent idea for someone who is unsure of what the field entails.

Although nursing schools do not require any prior healthcare work experience to be accepted into a nursing program, I highly recommend that if you're new to the profession, you should seriously consider gaining some familiarity around the health care environment. It would help with feeling overwhelmed on your first day of clinical and even your entry course work in nursing. This experience can be in the form of a hospital housekeeper (cleaning and maintenance person), patient transport, or even a nursing assistant, also known as a CNA — certified nurse's aide. Your newfound experience and knowledge of the healthcare environment in nursing is a crucial ingredient to your later success in the field. It's not uncommon at all for me to hear from new graduates who have received their state license, complaining that they just can't seem to land a job in the field — despite the shortage of nurses.

Well, this is primarily due to the fact that, although they have a nursing degree from a reputable school, and have successfully passed the NCLEX, they have zero experience in the field, and since the industry is quite competitive, their prospects for landing a job are significantly smaller than other students with practical experience. So it would behoove you during breaks between semesters to seek out opportunities to land some nursing/hospital experience. So having previous work experience in healthcare under your belt in some capacity is strongly advised. And if many of your peers who apply for the same jobs do have prior experience in healthcare and you do not, positions maybe offered to those individuals instead.

WHERE TO BEGIN?

First, my recommendation for new nurses is to start on a Medical Surgical unit first! Medical Surgical also known as Medical-Surgical nursing, is the structure and base of nursing. All other areas of nursing areas are considered specialties in nursing such as areas like ED, Emergency Department, ICU, Intensive Care Unit, or PACU, Post Anesthesia Care Unit, also known as the recovery room. Medical-Surgical is where a nurse can strategically learn to prioritize, organize, and manage their patient's care. Today's nurse patient ratio on a medical surgical unit can range from 1:4 (one nurse per four patients) to 1:7 (one nurse per seven). Or even more, depending on where you work. A mistake that a beginning nurse makes in their eagerness after graduating — in applying to areas such as Critical Care, Emergency Department (ED), Recovery Room (PACU), IR, Interventional Radiology, and other specialty areas.

New graduate nurses seem to have a stronger sense of energy and enthusiasm in the beginning of their nursing career. However, the above nursing areas mentioned are typically considered specialty areas and require a profound sense of critical thinking and ability to make decisions quickly. Such areas are special units and are not recommended for a new nurse to begin their nursing career. That is because these areas require critical thinking skills, which a new graduate does not have as a beginner nurse taking on their very first nursing job. Critical thinking skills take time to develop. Well-developed critical thinking skills afford a nurse the skills to quickly think on their feet in warranted situations.

OBTAIN A NURSING DEGREE FROM AN ACCREDITED SCHOOL

An aspiring new nurse has the option to obtain either an Associate's or Bachelor's degree in nursing. Associate degree programs typically take two years, while a bachelor's is typically a four-year program to complete. The associate degree program prepares students for entry-level nursing positions at a variety of venues, such as adult care facilities, hospitals, and other health-related establishments, as well as for a bachelor's degree in nursing, BSN degree.

The BSN is offered at colleges and universities, and prepares graduates to practice in all healthcare settings. It includes the study of research, leadership, healthcare informatics, and like me, healthcare policy. For the associate degree, job opportunities are becoming more and more scarce. This is because research reports that when nurses have the minimum of a bachelor education, the patient outcome is better.

Evidence of better nurses' performance and patient outcomes supports the baccalaureate for entry into nursing practice, according to "Preparing the Nursing Workforce for the Future," by Carol H. Ellenbecker, PhD, RN. Additionally, there is a significant difference between an associate degree in nursing (ADN) and a bachelor of science in nursing (BSN), with baccalaureate-prepared nurses demonstrating greater professional performance in the areas of communication skills, knowledge, problem solving, and professional roles.

Also, many employers such as hospitals are aiming to be Magnet hospitals, which equates nursing excellence and part of the application requirement for Magnet recognition is for a hospital to have a certain percentage of minimum baccalaureate nurses at its facility. Furthermore, where there is more emphasis on practical clinical experience outside the typical hospital setting because of the home health population, the associate degree nurse will eventually have to continue their education for either a bachelor's and/or a master's degree in nursing to remain competitive for career advancement.

Nursing school enrollment has become a booming business. Nursing program curricula come in all shapes and sizes. There is the traditional and Accelerated BSN program. The traditional nursing program of study is for someone who typically does not have a college degree and the curriculum is at a longer pace primarily because students are completing prerequisite courses. Although I have seen students who have completed an undergraduate degree in another field of study to go the traditional route, it's rare. The accelerated nursing programs of study are geared toward the student who has a bachelor's degree in another area of study. The program offers students a shorter duration of time of study to complete their degree. The word "accelerated" means the same as it sounds. Such programs move at an extremely fast pace, which is a pace fast enough that most people are not ready for. Unlike its counterpart, the BSN degree provides specific training in a more focused area of study such as leadership and communication.

Think about your finances, and if it may be more advantageous for you to attend a two-year program versus a four-year program, as the cost difference is rather significant. There's also the option of first completing the associate degree programs and subsequently transferring into the BSN program and supplementing this degree with scholarships and grants, which are great ways in financing this degree. There are many SONs, Schools of Nursing from colleges and universities beginning to partner with associate degree colleges, which is something that offers associate degree nurses the opportunities to continue their education at the university level once they have completed their associate degree. This is a viable option, as the credits from the associate degree do, in fact, transfer quite well into the BSN program at most accredited schools and also, this is to assist those students to assimilate into the nursing workforce into facilities meeting requirements for Magnet status.

As mentioned earlier, a nursing program's curriculum involves both theory and clinical. Theory can be defined as the lecture portion of the curriculum and the clinical course is the portion in which you will visit hospital sites and perform your clinical skills on real-life patients. This is the part which I find students lack in their skill ability, mostly because many programs focus heavily on theory but the clinical portion of the curriculum is equally important. The clinical part of the program is quite important (my bias because I teach clinical nursing). Many students will read and study an entire book in the theoretical framework and do well on exams, yet will be very uncomfortable when actually providing care to a real-life patient.

PASS THE STATE EXAMS & GET YOUR LICENSE

You heard me mention the NCLEX multiple times during your reading. All 50 states require a registered nurse to successfully pass the National Council Licensure Examination (NCLEX-RN). This exam is administered by the National Council of State Boards of Nursing, and can be a grueling process, as some students say, but with much preparation, and being a graduate from an accredited program, you will surely be granted registered nurse status for a state. The exam assesses an individual's minimum comprehensive knowledge and understanding of various topics in nursing (all that you should have learned from a quality nursing program). More specifically, the exam covers care management, health promotion skills, psychosocial and physiological integrity, preventative treatment abilities, and basic care to list a few.

Now the exam consists of you answering each multiple choice question (usually of four choices) and has since included your answers to be about how you would prioritize care while providing care to your patients. But it is impossible to say how the exam will alter in the future. Most students are anxious about the exam, but the good news is that nursing school is excellent preparation for successfully passing the NCLEX, especially if you attend a quality program and give yourself enough study preparation for the exam.

CHAPTER 5

Choosing the right nursing school: A how-to guide

When choosing a nursing program I suggest for you to do your homework! First and foremost, seek out and research nursing schools with programs at credible colleges and universities. I am quite surprised each time I hear of someone interested in attending nursing school that simply doesn't take the time to do due diligence and research the school that they are potentially interested in attending. After all, you're getting ready to spend a few years of your life and several thousand dollars on your nursing education. Wouldn't it be a good idea to do your research before making such an expensive decision?

Nursing schools offer students two curriculum programs of study consisting of traditional study or accelerated programs of study.

TRADITIONAL NURSING PROGRAM: The traditional nursing program is a popular option for a great number of students just out of high school. The program consists of either the Associate Degree in Nursing or four years BS/BSN. The Bachelor of Science in Nursing is an option depending on what degree you are seeking. One difference between the two is that it takes longer and would end up costing more in tuition in the four-year program. The ADN is offered by community colleges and hospital-based schools of nursing but the challenge is finding employment with an ADN degree, as most hospitals are requiring a minimum bachelor degree to be considered for a hire. But there is good news, if you choose to attend a school offering an ADN degree most community colleges have partnered with four-year colleges and universities to offer ADN graduates a chance to earn credits toward a BSN degree.

ACCELERATED NURSING PROGRAM: This program track is becoming increasingly popular among those who have an undergraduate, bachelor degree.

While the accelerated program is quite similar to the traditional program, the primary difference is that the duration is shorter, approximately 11-18 months to complete, designed for students who want to complete their degree in the fastest time possible. Accelerated baccalaureate programs offer the quickest route to licensure as a registered nurse (RN) for adults who have already completed a bachelor's or graduate degree in a non-nursing discipline. One of the best benefits to the accelerated program is finishing the degree faster but this concept comes with its own cost.

Accelerated baccalaureate programs accomplish programmatic objectives in a short time by building on previous learning experiences. Instruction is intense with courses offered full-time with no breaks between sessions. Students receive the same number of clinical hours as their counterparts in traditional entry-level nursing programs; it would be much more demanding of your time, which could add extra stress to you and may not benefit you in the long run.

Admission standards for accelerated programs are high, with programs typically requiring a minimum of a 3.0 grade point average (GPA) and a thorough pre-screening process. Identifying students who will flourish in this environment is a priority for administrators. Students enrolled in accelerated programs are encouraged not to work, given the rigor associated with completing degree requirements. Accelerated baccalaureate and master's programs in nursing are appropriately geared to individuals who have already proven their ability to succeed at a senior college or university. Having already completed a bachelor's degree, many second-degree students are attracted to the fast-track master's program as the natural next step in their higher education. Accelerated nursing programs are available in 46 states plus the District of Columbia and Puerto Rico. In 2012, there were 255 accelerated baccalaureate programs and 71 accelerated master's programs available at nursing schools nationwide and growing.

WHICH IS RIGHT FOR YOU?

From experience, depending on which group of students I am teaching, I find my encounters with the traditional students are in a not-so challenging mode, as opposed to the Accelerated Bachelor of Science in Nursing (ABSN) group of nurses. Specifically, I find traditional students to be less challenging in the clinical setting. The accelerated (ABSN) student seems to require more hand holding and guidance during clinical. Also, many of the traditional students are coming into the program with a health care background. They've worked or are working while attending nursing school.

My recommendation is for you to choose a program, when upon completion, you would receive at minimum a Bachelor of Science in Nursing Degree, as the industry is catering more toward individuals with higher academic credentials and more advanced training and experience, which the BSN offers. I would strongly advise you to spend a great deal of time researching the school's program history such as its graduation rate and national board exam pass rate (for first-time test takers), as such attributes are critical information to know. When you choose a school that looks like a good fit for you and your future career goals, I urge you to take a look at a number of factors such as:

COST: Nursing school is certainly not cheap, as is no acceptable amount of higher education, especially since the cost of tuition for higher education in America has skyrocketed over the past decade and currently the national student debt is over a trillion dollars. When considering the tuition cost for nursing school you should also factor books (ebook programs), clinical fees, all other necessary supplies and accessories, and other potential fees.

Also, there may be a situation requiring you to have room and board, which can be avoided if you choose a school close to home. Many students do not even realize the cost of tuition or how long it is going to take to pay off their student debt until after they've graduated and the bills start rolling in (six months post-graduation). When it comes to paying for tuition, there are many options for financing your nursing degree and it's not uncommon at all for students to take out student loans to help finance their tuition and even their living expenses while completing school. You should consider your options like a public program or a private program, as tuition factors are significantly different for these variables. In addition, you will want to consider whether you plan on attending nursing school in-state or out of state, as the price will significantly be different depending on that decision.

SCHOOL ENVIRONMENT: Road trip, anyone? After you've researched a variety of different nursing schools, my recommendation would be to narrow down your list, and if it is economically feasible, visit each of the schools and see them in person. After all, you're going to be investing a lot of money and spending the next few years of your life at school, so it's very important to make sure that you like the school, the location, and the campus. Visit the admissions office. Take a tour of the campus. Speak to other students on the campus in the program and pick their brains about their journey.

REVIEWS: Read the reviews and make sure they

align with your vision and career goals. When choosing a nursing school, one of the most vital things that you can do is to thoroughly research reviews on the school and its history. It's important for the voices of the current students to be heard. Do they like the school or don't they? Are they happy with their education or are they not? Are they learning real-life, hands-on nursing skills that they can apply in the field, or no? You'd be surprised at how many times I come across students who do not invest the time to read student reviews from the school they plan on attending only to later find out that they made the wrong decision. Reviews are powerful, and should certainly be utilized when you have the opportunity.

EXPERIENCE-BASED CREDIT: Over the years, I have had the pleasure of meeting nursing students that have had prior experience in the healthcare field, thus first being introduced to the field and subsequently pursuing a nursing degree after already being employed in the field. These students often have hands-on experience and have often been certified nursing assistants as well. If this applies to you, I would strongly recommend that you look into finding a nursing program that will offer you credits based on your prior healthcare experience. Certain nursing schools will, and others will not, all depending on a number of factors. If you have prior experience in the field, you might as well focus your search for nursing schools on the ones that are willing to recognize and reward your past experience. Ultimately, you will be required to take less courses before you graduate, which will behoove you in many ways (most notably: financially).

JOB PLACEMENT RATES: Make sure the school(s) you're thinking of attending have strong job placement rates for their graduating nurses, as some schools have much stronger job placement statistics than others, depending on a number of factors. While some of these factors may be out of the school's control (i.e. location, for instance), it is important to know what their job placement rates are so that you have a clear understanding of your chances of being employed upon graduation. Many schools (especially those with high job placement rates) will have these statistics posted on their website. Also, make sure that the schools tell you what kinds of jobs the graduates were able to receive.

Accreditation: It's important to make sure that your school is fully accredited by the National League for Nursing Accreditation Commission (NLNAC) or the Commission on Collegiate Nursing Education (CCNE). If the school in question is accredited by both, then that is even better. These bodies review the schools' policies, curricula, financial standing, boards of trustees, and instructors. Most nursing schools do, in fact, carry these accreditations and many of them clearly post it on their website and advertising brochure

NURSING SCHOOL IS NOT CHEAP!

As I've stated earlier, nursing school (just as any form of higher education) is not cheap, and any financial assistance will greatly behoove you and take a huge financial burden off your shoulders. Below are a few sites to reference for funding.

Places to Find Scholarships:
- www.nursingscholarship.us
- www.nursingsociety.org
- www.hrsa.gov/loanscholarships/scholarships/nursing
- www.scholarships.com

OTHER SOURCES FOR GRANTS & SCHOLARSHIPS

There are many other places to find scholarships, and the above list is only a small snippet of the information and resources that are available to you. Also, look into both grants and scholarships from the government, colleges, and private organizations. With the government, state governments, many times, will fund grants and scholarships for residents attending college in their state. As for colleges, sometimes the scholarships and grants they offer are merit-based or based on financial needs. Sometimes, they are actually a combination of the two.

PLACES TO FIND GRANTS

Applying for scholarships and grants will require you to fill out some basic financial aid forms such the Free Application for Federal Student Aid (FAFSA).

The basic steps are as follows:

1. Complete the FAFSA.

2. Find out what financial aid forms your college requires.

3. Research and apply for outside scholarships (this should be done well in advance of enrollment because scholarship funds go fast).

CHAPTER 6

A day in the life of a nursing student

So what is a typical day as a nursing student like anyway? Great question! Unfortunately, there is no clear-cut, black or white answer, as no two days as a nurse or a nursing student will ever be the same. Nursing school is an interesting blend of classroom work and clinical components. One of the most interesting facts is that there are some students who excel in classroom, yet they are uncomfortable performing physical assessments or administering medicine such as giving injections to their patients. Such skills are performed in the clinical portion of their studies, which a student will need to be successful in. Conversely, there are those who do not perform well on the classroom work, yet they are so comfortable and great with the patients during clinical.

Students should understand you must successfully receive a passing grade in both portions of the curriculum to be successful in the program. The truth is simple: To be a good nurse, you will need to have an excellent blend of being good in the classroom and the floor as well. Luckily, nursing schools are creative to teach you all there is to know about nursing. This helps in succeeding in structuring their programs. Generally, if you have a weakness in any area of the course work, the instructors will want to help strengthen your weakness in the most efficient way so that your once weakness becomes a strength and subsequently, you become a better nursing student in the process.

The advice from the students below will help give you an overall depiction of what you can anticipate as a nursing student: Myia T, a 2011 graduate, describes her experience as to what a typical week consists of.

She states: *"A typical week is as follows: 2 days of clinical and 3 days of classes and exams. I also work out daily. Working on campus job at desk and working one*

day every other week at the hospital. I also meet with study groups and study daily."
Myia T., RN, 2011 graduate

Although there is never a "standard" or "typical" day for any nursing student, Myia's experience is similar to many nursing students, as there is always a mix of clinical, classes, and exams. In addition, there is usually a substantial amount of time spent studying the material in order to ensure success on the exams. Some students spend many, many hours a week preparing for such exams, while others spend more time making sure they're nailing their clinical.

Megan, a 2015 graduate, describes her experience when she states: *"A typical week for myself is beginning the week with a checklist and making sure that I obey it. I write down assignments due, readings required that week, and studying. As graduation is getting near and boards will be just after that I have really started adding additional time to do questions and reviews in preparation for boards."*
Megan M., RN, 2015 graduate

Again, this is outstanding advice. While some people swear by doing checklists, other don't; however, I do believe that with the chaotic life of a nursing student, having a checklist that you can constantly refer back to in order to ensure that you're on target is a great idea and can certainly assist you in managing the workload. Another important thing that Megan mentioned is how important it is to prepare hard for the boards as graduation approaches. Many times, nursing students will not spend as much time studying as they should, and that usually doesn't end well. I am not going to lie to you: The nursing board exams are quite challenging, and there are very good nursing students who do not always pass on their first try. As long as you know what to expect on the exam, and you have diligence and make sure to study hard, you should be fine.

So the question remains: Is there really a typical day or a typical week? While each student's schedule varies greatly depending on a number of factors, Modestine shares her experiences as to what a typical week for her entails.

She states: *"In a typical week, you are in school or clinical 5 days out of 7. On a weekend, you're confined to a mosaic of assignments, group activities, research papers, studying and at times exams' preparations. In a typical weekday, I get up very early in the morning and prepare for a day mixed at times with clinical and on campus lectures. Although few days are blended with 'in class lectures' and clinical simultaneously, most days are filled with either one or the other. Overall, days and weeks can be very intense and exhausting!"*
Modestine, N., RN, 2015 graduate

In this instance, Modestine provides some of the most critical information of its kind. Essentially, she depicts the various aspects of the curriculum by showing that there are both classwork and clinical for five days, and then on the weekend there are both studying time and group work time. Yes, there will be a substantial amount of group work that is expected as well, but that's a good thing. Working with other nursing students is a great way for you to meet and network with your peers. In addition, the notion of working in a group provides you with the opportunity to work with other nurses and more importantly, to learn from those other nurses.

Take it from me: you can always learn from your peers.

What happens if you have a long commute to class? That's a great question, and luckily, technology has come to the rescue to make our lives easier.

Edyta, a 2014 graduate and working clinically states: *"As a nursing student I had two to three classes per week, so that meant I had to commute to school. While driving, I utilized recorded lectures and listen to them. I went to class took notes, came home and studied. I also had clinical twice a week. I left home about 5:30 am and came back around 8:00 pm, between a family and school I had to organize myself in order to conquer all. At night when everyone was asleep I studied until 1 or 2 a.m."*

This shows that Edyta would utilize her long commute time by listening to the lectures. This, as you can see, is an excellent use of time management. There are many students fortunate enough to live on campus, but there are also many students that, for some reason or another, have to commute a long distance to get to their school. If that happens to be you, utilizing your time by listening to lectures during your commute is an excellent way to multitask.

Deanne B., a 2015 graduate, shares her experience of what constitutes a typical day.

According to Deanne: *"A typical day for me was morning classes followed by work (part time), come home and study or do homework until I fall asleep. I would wake up and do it all over again the next day. I did not go out much with friends because I was trying to conserve money which is what allowed me to survive leaving my full-time job. I also did not have a lot of free time and time*

I did have, I felt like I needed to use wisely by reading."
Deanne B., RN, BSN, 2015 graduate

Deanne's profound statement reflects the life of a nursing student that shows the ultimate sacrifice: commitment. Deanne illustrates the fact that nursing school can often take its toll on your social life, and therefore, you may have to choose your priorities carefully. But it's not all treacherous work. Attending nursing school is also a great social experience and a chance to meet other future nurses and build your nursing network.

At this point, you may be asking yourself how to let go of some stress and unwind after a long day or classes, clinical, and studying. While each person has their own specific method of winding down after a long day, Lisa B., reiterates the importance of exercise for relieving stress.

She states: *"Studying all the time after class. It's really important to fit like at least 30 minutes to exercise every day because nursing school is really stressful."*
Lisa B., RN, 2015 graduate

Since it's a well-known fact that physical exercise releases endorphins and relieves stress that the body tends to carry around, it's no surprise that it would be advantageous for you to schedule at least 30 minutes a day to exercise and to clear your mind.

Riyona's experience is one that is filled with the typical class hours, followed by many hours of hitting the books to ensure that she's comprehended all of the necessary material for the exams.

She states: *"A typical day/week as a nursing student*

included waking up very early for my commute to school. I would then have classes for about 5 hours followed by studying for at least 2-6 hours afterward. Depending on the amount of homework, studying could last longer than 6 hours to make sure that all reading assignments were complete."

Riyona A., BSN, RN, 2014 graduate

HOW OFTEN DO YOU STUDY?

When conducting research for this book, I thought it was of the utmost importance to ask my students how many hours a day they devoted to studying for exams. Just as I suspected, many of the surveyed students responded that they study outside of class hours more intensely and for longer periods of time than they actually attend class. This is a vital ingredient to earning good grades and maintaining an edge on the strong competition that accompanies nursing school.

"I have classes 10 hours a week and study 35 hours a week or more."

Myia T., RN, 2011 graduate.

In this example, Myia spends over three times more time outside the classroom buried in her books, getting a leg up on the competition. For most students, there is an old academic saying that states something along the lines that if one spends 1 hour in the classroom, they should spend at least 2-3 hours studying.

Nursing school certainly follows this example, and Myia's schedule is living proof of that notion. When planning your class schedule, especially during your first year as a nurse, make sure to carve out enough time to follow this simple rule and you'll be well on your way to earning "A's": 1 hour in the classroom = 2-3 hours of outside studying. Edyta states that she spent 12-18 hours in class each week, and spent an additional 15-20 hours outside of class studying the material.

Occasionally, nursing students in their first year will take the most amount of classes and will sometimes wonder about burning out quickly. The truth is that your schedule may lighten up a bit toward the second year, so try and stay optimistic. Megan M., a 2015 graduate, shares her experience on this.

Megan states: *"Toward the beginning of the program I spent more time in class, up to 5 hours 2 days a week, and then additional lab hours. Now, I am currently just on campus twice a week for an hour and fifty minutes. I studied a lot! I was fortunate enough not to have to get a job during nursing school so I treated school like my job, which meant I was in the library for about 20-30 hours a week depending on the session."*
Megan M., RN, 2015 graduate

In this instance, Megan provides invaluable advice about the importance of acting like nursing school is your job. This is feasible for some students, and not so practical for others. If you have to work during nursing school and you cannot devote quite as much time studying that some of the other students, do not worry. As long as you make a strong effort to succeed and you continue with your dedication, you will do just fine.

"This Spring semester, I attended about 10 hours 'in class lectures per week' and study over 20 hours weekly."
Modestine, RN, 2015 graduate

Modestine clearly illustrates that she spends double her amount of class time outside studying to ensure she has the material locked-down for test day.

"In the beginning of nursing school I took the most classes (4 times weekly, clinical 1 time weekly 12hr). Towards the end of the program I had class twice a week and clinical once a week typically (12 hr). Each class was usually 3 or 4 hours long. I also took an online class almost each session. I spent about 2hrs a day studying."
Deanne B., RN, BSN, 2015 graduate.

"9 hrs. a week in class. At least 50 hrs. week studying especially for Medical-Surgical and Critical care."
Lisa B., RN, 2015 graduate

THE TRUTH ABOUT CLINICAL

One of the most common questions I hear from first-year nursing students or those considering a career in the nursing field are questions relating to clinical. Clinical can be tough, but really it's only what you make it to be. Clinical is essentially the intersection where theoretical knowledge and hands-on training and experience come together. When these two aspects come to a life, a great nurse is formed. There is no such thing as the great nurse who only knows theory and isn't good in a "hands on" sense, just as there is no such thing as a nurse who is great with patients but lacks the theoretical framework that is taught during classroom lectures and the textbooks. The two come together to make someone a great nurse, thus the importance of performing well in clinical is quite high. That being said, clinical has an interesting reputation. This section will help facilitate your knowledge of clinical and what to expect when you begin the clinical portion of your education and training.

Myia shares her experience by saying the experience was frightening — something I hear all too often.

She states: *"It was scary. There is a difference between reading about being a nurse and actually doing it. The staff was very welcoming and the patients seemed excited about having a student nurse to help them. Clinical was not what I had expected. I thought it would be a little more hands-on."*
Myia T., RN, 2011 graduate

Myia's experience is quite typical, as most students don't always realize the gap between the theoretical knowledge and the actual hands-on experience that you will gain by actually performing the things you previously learned about. Some students are naturals at this and excel right from the beginning. With other students, they seem more uncomfortable and timid in the beginning, but they eventually find their touch and it becomes easier and easier for them to care for their patients.

On the contrary, I've also seen students who struggled a bit with the theoretical classroom aspect of nursing school, but seemed to be naturals when it came to the clinical portion of their education. It really all boils down to the person, but I've found that those who enter nursing school with some kind of prior hospital or volunteer experience are the ones that are the most successful during their clinical.

They seem comfortable and unfazed by treating patients. They feel comfortable and confident about stepping in and taking care of a patient.

Edyta says that she was both nervous and excited at the same time, which is quite common for most students.

She states: *"The clinical instructor was great, she made sure we learn as much as we can during every clinical day. Unfortunately location and availability of hands on experience was not there all the time. I think we could have had a better location."*

One thing to remember about fear is this: Do not be afraid of clinical. They are simply a part of being a successful nurse; therefore, you should look forward to them because you cannot be a good nurse unless you nail the clinical aspect of the craft as well. I know it may be a bit frightening at first, but you will be more comfortable before too long. Megan M., describes her experience as most nursing students do: petrifying!

She states: *"My first day of clinical was petrifying! I remember going into the patient's room and stumbling with my words, and I specifically remember attempting to get a blood pressure on a heavier patient and being way too cautious with moving the patient's arm because I didn't want to hurt her."*

As a nursing instructor, I hear these stories all the time, and let's say, it's perfectly normal to be a somewhat anxious one, because now you're with real patients and their care will be in your hands. I have seen many nursing students fear that they will hurt a patient while giving them a shot or taking their blood, and because of this fear, they act unconfident and perform the task not as well as they could. Many times, this is just a small fear and once the student has more experience with various patients, they will get over it and it will be a non-issue. Megan also shares her experiences about her medicine and surgical clinical and critical care clinical, which were more challenging than she thought. She felt as if she was being pushed beyond her limits. She states,

"My Med-Surg. clinical and Critical Care clinical were beyond what I expected. I was pushed to do things at the time beyond what I felt I was capable of doing, but it has built my confidence up and has allowed me to believe in myself. Other clinical settings were disastrous, and I truly tried to find a silver lining, but it's still hard for me to look back and outweigh the positives to the negatives."
Megan M, RN, 2015 graduate.

EXPLORING A TYPICAL DAY IN THE LIFE OF A NURSING STUDENT

One of the most common questions I receive from nursing students is how to cope with the inevitable stress that a nursing student faces. If you're feeling a bit overwhelmed by the rigorous academic work, that is expected. The best way to anticipate the stress is to consider a typical day of a nursing student, so you have an idea of the demands of the task before you. Below is a typical day in the life for a nursing student on a clinical site. Note the observations of the student, as these provide fodder for consideration.

A PREVIEW OF A DAY AS A NURSING STUDENT

(Medical Surgical nursing clinical rotation by a Chamberlain College student):

4:00 a.m.: I'm awake.

5:00 a.m.: Out the door.

7:00 a.m.: At the clinical site, lateness cannot be afforded. Two late arrivals equal an absence. Two absences are a failure of the class. A bad thing about some nursing schools is as long as they provide you a clinical site, which can be in a 50-mile radius of the campus, it is your responsibility how you arrival to your assigned clinical site. Now that you know, it's best you become aware of the clinical sites that your school has.

7:30 a.m.: Assigned two patients and patient care begins: Vital signs obtained, cleaning, moving, positioning, transferring, and feeding are all components of care for a med-surg. patient. It requires grit and patience to do it appropriately. While doing your job appropriately, you also have to consider your own posture and most hospitals today provide nurses with lift devices to use when manipulating their patients. The rates of back pain among nurses are to be considered. This is the hardest part of the job, I believe. The other critical part is medication administration which, 99.9% of the time, you will be right if you follow proper protocols of administering medication (the 5Rs: the right patient, the right drug, the right dose, the right route, and the right time, which you will learn in nursing pharmacology. Some facilities have 7Rs. Practice calculating medical dosages.

On this fateful day, I donned my glove, ready to dive in and begin accruing nursing experience. I have been assigned to an incontinent patient who soils himself regularly and requires changing to keep clean and dry and yes, this is the responsibility of the nurse.

9:00 a.m.: When I was done, I felt as though I had achieved a feat, and as I got back to the hallway, my professor asked why I was still on one patient and hadn't gotten to looking up my drugs at all. I felt slightly bad that I wasn't on schedule, but I was absolutely satisfied that I took my time taking care of my patient and the patient was grateful for it. For if I were in the same position, I would appreciate someone taking good care of me rather than doing a finicky job and just jumbling things together.

Here is where managing and prioritizing care could have helped this student.

10:00 a.m.: Medication administration.

11:00 a.m.: All day long, there will continually be some sort of cleaning to do, or dressing, feeding, assessment, in addition to medication administration.

12:00 p.m.: A break of about an hour was given.

1:00 p.m.: Back on the floor and afternoon medications were given, along with other patient care.

4:00 p.m.: By the time I left at 4 p.m. and arrived home at 6 p.m., I could only rush to lie on my bed, considering the back-breaking pain and weariness I was overwhelmed with.

As a nursing student, I've learned that direct patient care is not my forte even though I currently provide the best care to my patients and will continue to do so.

If the money that comes with nursing attracts you, but you find the direct contact aspect of nursing distasteful and you're planning to work in a hospital, please, please, take your time to find something else with more pay, because you'll be quite miserable and the money received will never suffice. Another good thing is, nursing is not limited to direct patient contact, but direct care is mostly what is available. Starting out with direct patient care is never a bad idea.

If your heart of compassion is all there is that drew you to nursing, and you have the strength to care for people, you are what the patients want, and you will feel fulfilled helping them.

•

Perhaps the final line of this student's testimony is the most compelling, and the one that acts as the glue that holds all your career aspirations together, as it ties back to the core of all people thinking of becoming nurses: compassion. The last line stated, "If your heart of compassion is all there is that drew you to nursing, and you have the strength to care for people, you are what the patients want, and you will feel fulfilled helping them." This is one of the most true things that I have ever, personally, read, which is why this is vital to be included.

Here illustrates a day in the life of a nursing student on a clinical day, one that is quite busy as all nursing students tend to be. Do you think you could handle a schedule such as this one? Are you prepared? Hopefully, the answer is, "YES!"

CONFIDENCE IS KEY

Keep in mind that although you will succeed in the end, the first day or even the first few weeks into your clinical can be very challenging, and it is very common for students to feel a certain level of anxiety in relation to the added stress. But remember always demonstrate confidence! Modestine's experience outlines this overwhelming feeling.

She states: *"The first day of clinical, I felt like I was at the fork of the road with one pathway exhibiting anxiety and an overwhelmed feeling and the other pathway filled with eagerness and determination to learn. I will say that clinical did meet my expectation because my previous nursing assistant experience helped me anticipate some patient care puzzles and facilitated my transition. I must say however that moving from the dummy in the simulation lab to a real patient brought some anxiety and fear."*
Modestine, RN, 2015 graduate

My first day of Med-Surg. clinical I was nervous because it was going to be the first time that we were going to get to fully experience nursing in the hospital setting. We would be passing meds as well as working with IVs and assisting with other procedures. At this point in the program we did not know enough to see the whole picture, which made it very intimidating. As the session continued, we were able to quickly put the pieces together and everything started to make sense.

"Clinical was much more than I expected. It is very difficult to balance the workload in the beginning. I almost felt like it was an overload of material the very first

week. It is only because I was taking two other classes and everything was completely new. After getting over the shock I was amazed at how clinical helped me to see what I was actually absorbing and it allowed me to see and experience many of the things we talked about in class first-hand. I did not know that I would get the opportunity to visit other units in the hospital, and get to do as much as we were able to do. I also realized that the more you put into clinical the more you will get out of it. In some cases you may even land an internship or job when you finish school."

Deanne B., RN, BSN, 2015 graduate

"I was so nervous probably because I didn't want to mess up in front of clinical instructor so I was very nervous because I didn't want to look dumb. So I remember stuttering a lot when doing my assessment on a patient. I don't think clinical is realistic because you only get 1 patient but most hospitals have 5-7 patients at a time so it's important to patients in a realistic situation like a real nurse."

Lisa B. RN, 2015 graduate

Lisa's experience rings true to so many other soon-to-be nurses. The amount of nervous tension in your body can be a bit overwhelming, yet it can work to your advantage as long as you let it. For instance, being a little nervous can be a good thing, as being nervous will allow you to focus and pay attention to what you're doing. You'll be more focused on what you are doing, and ultimately, the patient will receive better care as a result.

"My first day of clinical was very scary. I remember feeling so nervous, but very excited at the same time.

I wanted to learn as much as possible, but not mess anything up because this was the 'real thing.' Overall the experience was OK. I believe it could have been a better experience if the clinical site and preceptor were more conducive to my learning experience."

Riyona A., BSN, RN, 2014 graduate

If I had to tally up the number one emotion that most students tell me when describing their experience, I would inevitably say fear trumps all other emotions.

Jennifer states: *"My first day was very frightening. Before then I had only been in a nursing home type setting. I really didn't know what to expect. It was very busy telemetry unit. It took time on how to schedule my tasks, look for equipment/ supplies, and overall interact with the patients. During this phase, I typically shadowed the RN scheduled to those patients. It was also very challenging because I didn't obtain the basic hands-on skills prior."*

Jennifer R., BSN, RN, 2014 graduate

Make sure to keep your expectations in check. One of the most ironic things when speaking with students about clinical is the common misconception that students seem to have about what clinical actually entails. It seems that somewhere along the way, they have been taught a barrage of common myths.

Jennifer R. states: *"I really didn't know what to expect during clinical. The books can only teach you so much. I realized there were different expectations from units, preceptors, and the staff on the floors. Some RNs were more than willing to teach, others just wanted to check in with us if something was wrong. Even though it was a very busy hospital, I am glad to have had that*

exposure at such a critical time in a nursing student's curriculum. MedSurg was the backbone to the rest of my clinicals throughout the program."
Jennifer, R., BSN, RN, 2014 graduate

Listen to what Jennifer said: *"Books can only teach you so much."*

This invaluable advice comes from a nursing student that has seen the substantial dichotomy that lies between the theoretical knowledge that one can obtain from books in comparison to the hands-on experience that can only be obtained through actually rolling up your sleeves and getting down to the nitty gritty. Shockingly, there are still some students that are overly confident before they have ever seen a patient in person. Some of them have the textbook portion nailed, yet they don't realize just how difficult clinicals are. It is during this time that many of them drop their egos and begin learning how to "really" be a successful nurse: by making sure the patient is number one, always.
Some students find employment rather quickly, oftentimes within just weeks of graduating and passing the state board examinations.

"I graduated the end of October 2014, took my boards the first week of December, and accepted employment by January 15, 2015."
Jennifer R., BSN, RN, 2014 graduate

Jennifer's story seems to ring true with many nursing graduates. Luckily, she made contacts during nursing school and did an excellent job networking with her peers. As a result, she was able to land a full-time employment position just shortly after she finished passing the board exams.

Here, the graduates have expressed their first experience of their hospital clinical. In reading these comments one would not find nursing school positive. Such expressions were initial feelings the students had, mostly because they did not know what to expect and or had no experience in a hospital environment. Again, this is why some experience within a hospital environment is crucial and highly recommended prior to beginning your nursing school journey.

Additionally, although each graduate expressed some fear, they were able to overcome such feelings, and remained focused to complete their clinical experience. Each academic term required another clinical rotation related to the subject of study. According to the graduates, each clinical got better as well as their skills. I must add that each of these students graduated and are successful, practicing nurses and you can also do the same.

When writing this book, having a section that clearly illustrated the "truth" about the clinical portion of a nurse's education was one of the most important pieces. In essence, there is a plethora of rumors that float around about what clinicals really are, how often you'll be engaged in them, and how they really shape your academic experience. It is my sincere wish that you will find all of the stories helpful, but that this will not scare you away from enrolling in nursing school.

HOW TO SURVIVE YOUR FIRST SEMESTER TERM OF NURSING SCHOOL

Although it would be ideal if every nursing student knew what to expect on their first day of class, then there wouldn't be a need for this book. That is certainly not the case, as you will soon see once your first day arrives and classes officially begin.

The purpose of this section is to provide you with all of the information you'll need to survive your first day of class.

Chamberlain College of Nursing surveyed some of their students on what advice they would give to a student on their first day. Their answers captured every angle of what a successful student would need to know.

Their responses are as follows:

• Be prepared for the hardest, scariest, most rewarding day of your life.

• Print your syllabus and follow along week by week. Look ahead and cross off as you go and before you know it, eight weeks will be done. — Cari C.

• Treat your first class as important as your last class. Stay strong throughout every class so when your last class truly comes you are fully ready to ace your boards. — Alyssa V.

• Ask for help early if you need it. Take a deep breath. — Pam B.

• Don't be discouraged if you don't do well on your first test, you'll know you have to work harder to keep moving forward. — Edwin S.Jr.

• Be confident and courageous. You can do anything you have your heart set on. — Charmaine K.

• Stay organized! — Soroya B.

• It's okay to be a little scared. Study hard and

don't be afraid to ask for help from your instructors. — Melanie D.

• Reach out for tutor and writing help. Use that library access; link for formatting references on right side, so use it! — Kathleen D.

• Don't get behind on your reading. Give yourself time to study to avoid cramming it all in. Get a good night's sleep before exam day. — Donabel P.

•

Much of the advice provided by these students is invaluable. That being said, there truly is not a foolproof way of preparing, as each and every day is different. Part of being an excellent nurse is being able to embrace each and every day with an open heart and an open mind. There is nothing I can do or say to you that will prepare you for the journey that lies ahead. It is a glorious journey, but certainly, there are bumps in the road that you will encounter.

CHAPTER 7

How to survive the NCLEX exam: Everything you need to know

So, you've done it! You've officially graduated from the rigorous, grueling curriculum of a nursing school. However, you're still not legally allowed to be a practicing nurse until you successfully complete your respective state's NCLEX exam. I understand your pain. It feels as if you've accomplished something amazing by completing nursing school, but you still cannot fully relax until the stress and anxiety of completing the NCLEX has been lifted from your trembling shoulders. Fear not. While most students and soon-to-be nurses are terrified of such an exam, the exam sounds more intimidating than it actually is. The good news is that as long as you are well-prepared and follow the advice within this chapter, you will have a very strong chance at surviving the exam.

HOW TO PREPARE FOR THE EXAM

Here is a compelling list of the best way to successfully prepare for the exam:

• Don't wait!: Some nurses finish school and they immediately feel that it's necessary to take some time off and reward themselves with some time to de-stress their minds by taking a relaxing vacation or simply taking a "stay-cation." While this is not the worst option, many studies show that waiting to take the NCLEX exam is usually not a good idea. Some nurses finish school and are very eager to begin working, thus they schedule the exam almost immediately after they graduate. This is the best, most feasible option, as the course material is still the freshest in your mind. In addition, there is really no reason to delay taking the exam.

• Study Study Study!: Now this may seem quite obvious and I am not trying to state obvious facts, but you would be surprised at the number of students that do not spend a considerable amount of time in their studies. There is no magic number of how long or how much you should study for the NCLEX in any given time period; however, as a general rule of thumb, I would recommend allowing yourself a solid three or even four weeks of intense, focused studying before taking the exam.

FORM A STUDY PLAN FOR NCLEX

You need to figure out a game plan for NCLEX and how you are going to cover your bases and hit on everything you've learned. Get an overview book and do as many practice questions as you can to prepare for the test of your life. Make a schedule for studying. Form a study group. You should be channeling all of your time and effort over the next few weeks into the NCLEX exam.

• Prep classes: Is taking an NCLEX preparatory class a good idea, you ask? Well, it certainly isn't a bad idea. There are certain well-known exam preparatory classes offered by Kaplan, and a few other select brands that guarantee they have high-pass ratios. Taking a preparatory class, in my humble opinion, is an excellent idea; however, it may not always be feasible.

I'm not going to mislead you: Preparatory classes are certainly not cheap, and that is the primary reason why some students shy away from taking them. Some students can afford them and others cannot. If you can afford them without breaking the bank, then I would suggest giving a preparatory class a shot. You will meet and network with other nursing students and you will have the chance to study with them outside of class as well. If you are a bit strapped for cash, please don't feel any additional anxiety by thinking that preparatory classes are mandatory, because they're not. As long as you did well in nursing school and you are a motivated, self-disciplined student, you shouldn't have a problem passing the exam.

AVOIDING DISTRACTIONS

Avoid all distractions when studying: Distractions can kill even the most motivated of students when they're trying to cram for the NCLEX exam; therefore, it is vital that you eliminate those distractions to the very best of your ability. Below is a list that I've compiled on the very best ways to eliminate distractions, since distractions inhibit one's ability to study.

- Turn off everything: Have you ever imagined what it would be like to live in a world without cell phones, social media, or technology? Well, you should find out when you're preparing for the NCLEX exam because ALL of your technology and outlets to the world should be turned off at this time. Turn off your phone, iPad, Kindle, laptop, TV, computer, and STUDY. A good method for fighting the temptation to check your phone or for social media updates when studying is to shut off all devices and them remove the batteries from them or have someone hide them from you until you're done studying for the day. It might sound funny, but it truly works! I should also mention that there are no exceptions to this rule. If you have a compelling, insatiable urge to check your phone or your social media pages, it is important that you teach yourself to refrain from doing this until you've successfully completed your studying. It does take both time and discipline but in the end, you'll be glad you did.

• Find what works for you: Everyone who has ever studied for anything in their life has an opinion on the best way to study, but rather than filling your head with all of their ideas and advice, you should find whatever works best for you and then exclusively stick to that method of studying. Some people don't mind a noisy environment when they study, so they prefer to study in local cafes. For others, the notion of silence is similar to a golden virtue, and if the room is not completely silent, they find themselves easily annoyed and unable to study. Some people find that studying for several hours a day is the best way to go.

QUESTIONS AND ANSWERS ABOUT THE EXAM

Q: What are the common test questions? How can I prepare for them if I don't know exactly what the test is going to ask?

A: You are never going to know exactly what test questions are going to be asked, but there are many great resources out there for helping you prepare and providing you with a strong background for answering the questions correctly. That being said, the NCLEX includes case scenarios, correct options, and distracter options. There is a great percentage of priority questions.

Q: What happens if I did not pass the exam?

A: For students who were unsuccessful in passing the exam, you will receive a Diagnostic Profile which provides information about strengths and weaknesses in certain test areas. In addition, you will be able to see how close you were to passing. And you'll have an opportunity to retake the exam after a lapse of time, and of course, for an additional fee.

•

This chapter helped to prepare you for your licensure exam. Now that you have an idea of what to expect, you can determine if the stress of preparing for and taking the NCLEX exam is something you can handle.

Next up: Let's talk money!

CHAPTER 8

Show me the money: Salary for new nurses and seasoned nurses

Although I have been spending a great deal of time driving the point home that those entering the nursing field simply for the money are making the wrong decision, it's important to provide the most recent data on what kind of salary a new nurse and even a well-seasoned nurse can expect. After all, you need to make sure that you can support yourself and/or your family working as a nurse, and the good news is that you can!

PAYDAY: I always tell my students nursing will be good to you if you are good to nursing. Recent nursing school graduates are happily enjoying some of the nation's highest starting salaries among their peers in other industries. Salaries do vary from state to state, so do your homework when you begin your employment search. According to results of a 2012 AORN salary and compensation survey, job title, education level, certification, experience, and geographic region, affect a nurse's compensation.

Nurses can attain a salary where they can comfortably take care of their family, but they certainly have to work for it. A career as a nurse takes hard work and long hours, and many nurses have to make sacrifices from time to time when it comes to their work schedule and hours. It's a common myth held by some people that nurses have easy schedules because they are only expected to be at the hospital for three days in a work week. That's three 12-hour shifts at one work place. The cold, hard truth is that nurses work very, very hard and long hours in those three days. A nurses' workday can be action-packed, so packed that nurses rarely have the time to eat lunch or dinner during those shifts, and often do not even go to the bathroom (that's a running joke, but so true). Some nurses can spend the entire shift on their feet, thus leaving them very tired at the end of a grueling 12-hour shift. Typically, after a 12-hour day, I am exhausted, and I have very little time to do much after work. Usually it's home, maybe eat, and head to bed to prepare for the next day. In addition to three 12-hour shifts in a week, many nurses pick up extra shifts.

A nurse's salary can vary tremendously depending on where you decide to take up employment. Working at a hospital (not a clinical) a nurse can easily earn a median income upwards of $56,000 to $98,400. The average nurse in the United States is currently earning at minimum $69,790 and the average hourly wage of a registered nurse is $33.55. These averages, of course, are based on the fact that a registered nurse may make more or less than these figures due to the location, experience, and other factors like being armed with certification in a specialty, and most importantly, degree earned. All of these factors can provide a nurse high earning power.

GEOGRAPHICAL LOCATION: If you currently think that where you choose to practice nursing doesn't have an effect on how much money you'll be earning, then I urge you to think again. There are reports that a registered nurse's salary is highly determined by geographical location. Living on the West Coast, particularly in the state of California, for instance, means being in an area where nurses are the highest paid.

The average salary of a registered nurse working in Sacramento has a number of $108,340, Oakland, California is $121,040 and San Jose, California is $123,190 annually. Next is San Francisco where an average salary of a registered nurse can be a whopping $127,670 that was in 2014, when an hourly wage for a registered nurse was $47.31. Do your homework folks and you'll get an eye-opener of the current numbers from state to state. As you can see, nurses quite frankly, can earn a healthy income but it takes skills choosing employment. So please take time when planning this very important task. Some people may feel the money is worth it; others may decide there are easier or less stressful ways to earn money, which you will personally decide for yourself.

CHAPTER 9

The nitty-gritty of finding work

L anding a job is a pretty big goal of any nursing student. After all, all of the studying, test-taking, and work have been leading to this. So let's look at what you need to do to give yourself the best chance of landing just the job you want.

DO PREPARE A RESUME

You're going to need a resume to send out to people who are going to hire you, and it has probably been a long time since you updated yours. Now you can include nursing school, any volunteer work you've done, and any work as a CNA in a facility. Your resume is a very important tool in your job search and it is important that you spend a substantial amount of time on it in an effort to truly show your accomplishments and highlight your career path.

There are many talented nurses out there that do not have strong resumes, perhaps because they're not strong writers, or because they are unfamiliar with how to write an eye-catching resume, or simply they won't spend the money to have it professionally done. There are many legitimate, online resume services that you can turn to. In addition, the career and/or guidance counselor at your nursing school should be able to offer you some assistance here.

GET AN INTERVIEW OUTFIT: DRESS APPROPRIATELY FOR SUCCESS

It is important to look your best when you go on interviews for nursing jobs. While this is usually common knowledge, not everyone follows it. You should have something that is business appropriate, fits well, and makes a good impression on Human Resource and nurse managers alike. Make sure what you're wearing is clean, crisp, and unwrinkled. Remember that you only have one chance to make a good first impression on a hiring manager. Despite what anyone tells you, it does matter how you're dressed, and people will judge you. Also, warrants mentioning: If you have them, please cover up any tattoos and piercings; consider not wearing nose and lip rings to an interview. And please do not wear jeans to your interview.

FIND A MENTOR TO ASSIST WITH INTERVIEW QUESTIONS

Get yourself a good mentor, perhaps a former instructor (I've mentored countless students), a close peer, or a colleague who can assist and guide you on this path of securing employment. Another important aspect of getting ready for hire is to learn interview questions and the best, most effective answers to those questions. Do your research. You're going to want to ace the interview, so remember that this is critical!

THE INTERVIEW

Toward the end of the interview, don't forget to smile, shake the hand of the person interviewing you, and most of all thank them for their time. In addition, I always advise students that they should ask for that person's business card and send a follow-up "thank you" response to them approximately 24 hours after the interview. Most candidates do not do that; therefore, sending a follow-up letter of that thank you for the interviewer for giving their time and speaking with you of the positions goes a long way and will most likely set you apart from other candidates.

HOW LONG WILL IT TAKE FOR YOU TO FIND A JOB AFTER GRADUATING AND PASSING THE STATE BOARDS?

If I had a dollar for every time a nursing student asked me how long after graduating before they would likely find a job, I'd have enough dollars to retire, buy a beach house off the Pacific coast of California (what I so want to do), and never work another day in my life. Although it's a legitimate question to ask, there really is no clear-cut answer, as all students in various scenarios begin working in different times following completing their degree. While not all students find employment within the same time frame, generally speaking, it should not take more than one to three months.

In fact, it's very common for students to be employed before they graduate. I have had many students over the years become employed in a hospital or doctor's office a few weeks or months before their graduation date, contingent on them successfully finishing school. The good news is that the nursing field has proven itself time and time again to be a recession-proof industry, which is only one of the many benefits to being a nurse.

Here, a new graduate found employment in *"two months, but through someone I knew."*
Myia T, RN, 2011 graduate

On average, two months is a very reasonable amount of time to be in the job market. Again, there are many different factors that play into an individual's ability to land employment upon graduating, and those factors will vary greatly from student to student.

Deanna B. shares her story.

She states: *"I worked for a home health agency as a CNA during nursing school. They hired me as a nurse after I passed my boards. I went to a career fair at Mercy Hospital prior to taking my boards and I interviewed for a position in the ICU. The nursing manager hired me pending me passing my state boards, but it took so long for my license to show, they gave the position away. I spoke with HR and interviewed for Neuro/Tele and I was hired in that department. I begin orientation May 18, 2015. I took my state boards April 6th and graduated end of February."*

Deanna B., RN, BSN, 2015 graduate

Edyta shares her experience and stated that she graduated in October, took the state board in December, and found employment right away.

She proclaims: *"Easy. I decided to take few months off due to my family. I did not even apply to any jobs. My friend from nursing school was working in the hospital she called me that a unit manager ask her if she knows someone who would like to work on oncology unit and has amazing work ethics. She called me, and I went for an interview. I was lucky enough to get the job offer on the spot."*

How great would it be to simply be given a job offer right on the spot? Pretty cool, huh? It's possible, as you can see with Deanna's experience.

So, there you have it. Some students have jobs before

they graduate, and others take a bit longer. The truth is that there has always been and remains a strong demand and a shortage of qualified nurses, thus there will certainly be many opportunities for you finding work upon completing your degree. Yes, even in this treacherous economy, the nursing industry is booming.

HOW DIFFICULT WILL IT BE?

For the most part, being hired as a nurse should be a piece of cake. One possible challenge is if you have no experience at all in the healthcare field. Once again, if you haven't worked as a CNA through nursing school, you should consider working as one during the time between nursing school and taking the NCLEX. Not only will it give you experience, but it will also help you get a foot in the door in a potentially hiring facility. One of the most interesting comments I've received about the difficulty in finding work was from Myia, a 2011 graduate, who is now gainfully employed in the field.

Myia stated that it was *"Challenging. No one wanted to hire or train a new grad."*

Please take this advice with a grain of salt, as she is not saying that there are not opportunities available for new graduates. She is merely stating that the employment industry in nursing is a demanding field and is more competitive now than years ago because of the influx of new graduates and the overwhelming enrollees into nursing schools. Megan's experience was quite different than Myia's.

She states: *"Fortunately, I have many family members*

in the medical field, so I utilized my resources and landed myself a wonderful externship opportunity on my dream location, labor & delivery."
Megan M., RN, 2015 graduate

Hearing this made my day. It's stories like these that I love hearing because they show that someone can land their dream job right out of school. Fortunately, for Megan's sake, she had a strong family network in the medical field, and she leveraged those resources into landing her a job. Yes, it could be a matter of who you know in the field. The most important piece of advice I can offer here is to build your network during nursing school so that you have contacts and possibly employment opportunities when you graduate. Don't be afraid to network or make connections, as that is how to land a job in our current economic downturn.

I always ask students after they land a job how they did it and what kind of tactics they would recommend to future graduates. In today's contemporary social networking phenomenon, most of them recommend LinkedIn and other sites geared toward nursing professionals. While all of those options are good, I recently spoke with Deanna B., who offered some profound insight on how she landed her first job after graduating. She mentioned something that most students completely overlook: a career fair. I know the notion of a career fair is great for nurses today, as the meeting of people face-to-face still goes a long way.

Deanna states: *"I found it easy to find employment only because I went to the career fair. I feel that if I had not gone, it would have taken me so much longer to find a position in a hospital. Many positions require you to have a license in hand in order to apply and the process takes*

a long time. I utilized the career services office often. Emily helped me with my resume as well as preparing for my interviews ahead of time. Each time I interviewed I was offered the position. Her advice really helped a lot."
   Deanna B., RN, BSN, 2015 graduate

Job fairs at community hospitals are a good choice to attend. Networking with various hospitals, doctor's offices, and other nursing professionals in the area does help as well. Although most of the networking that occurs in today's technologically advanced internet world tends to occur through social networking websites, I can honestly say that there is something timeless about actually networking with people face-to-face. There is something to be said for an applicant that puts in the time to meet and network with people during a career fair and in-person.

ORIENTATION CONSIDERATIONS

- What is the level and depth of orientation?
- Will more orientation time be granted if I feel I need it?
- Will my orientation take place during the shift I will be working?
- Is there a mentorship program?
- What are your expectations of new hires during their first six months on the job?
- Describe typical first-year assignments.
- What qualities do your most successful nurses possess

WHAT IS REQUIRED OF A NEW NURSE UPON GETTING HIRED?

Today, for hiring purposes, many medical facilities have a minimum requirement of a baccalaureate degree at their respective facilities. This is becoming more and more common, partially because higher academic credentials are used to distinguish candidates, given the competitive nature of the job market, and healthcare facilities are obtaining Magnet status. Also, when it comes to resumes, hire a professional to help you construct your resume. Students often scoff at this notion, yet there are thousands of professional resume writers out there, and the vast majority of them do excellent work. Also, human resources searches for specific attributes during the hiring process, specifically, if you have a membership with a nursing organization and if you have any previous healthcare experience.

A LITTLE SOMETHING ABOUT PROFESSIONAL ORGANIZATIONS

Because nursing is a profession and not just a "job," being a member of a professional organization demonstrates the fact that you take your nursing career seriously, which is one more attribute that sets you apart from your competition. Another way to distinguish yourself from the crowd is to join a nursing organization of your choice — preferably an organization specific to the area of specialty, which you work; for example AMSN, Academy of Medical-Surgical Nurses, or AACN, American Association of Colleges of Nursing. If you work on a medical-surgical unit you should also become a member of the national organization, and become involved in its local chapter.

SO, YOU'RE HIRED! NOW WHAT?

So you've graduated school, you've passed boards, you've applied to jobs, you've interviewed, and you've just accepted your first job! Congratulations! This is a very exciting time for you. Although it is very exciting, it can also be a bit confusing. Luckily, reading this book will aid you in the process as much as possible and hopefully take away some of the pre-first day stress that you may be feeling. You can breathe a sigh of relief knowing that your nursing education has well prepared you for what's to come.

ORIENTATION

When first becoming a nurse, the orientation process is one that is rapidly changing as each year passes by. When I first began nursing years ago, my orientation process was at minimum 3 and 6 months depending on how well you were progressing through the process and also the nursing unit you trained on. I thoroughly enjoyed the extensive orientation, as I felt like I was learning more in orientation than I had in school and that rigorous training was facilitating me to become the best possible nurse I was capable of becoming. Although that was my experience, orientation is now a far cry from what it used to be.

Today, you will be lucky if you can find a healthcare facility still standing that is willing to offer you a 3-week orientation, let alone 3-6 months! That, essentially, is due to a lack of financial support and rudimentary level economics. After all, healthcare is a business, and I certainly don't need to convince you that everything in this world seemingly boils down to economics, and so does nursing. I soon realized something very important after I began working in healthcare: Economics is a ubiquitous feature of our lives. Even in healthcare. It was like that back when I started in the profession and more certainly it is like that today.

A DAY IN THE LIFE OF A NURSE

Throughout the entire course of this book, you've been learning about deciding on whether attending nursing school is a good option for you or not, you've been learning about how to select the right nursing school for you, you've been learning how to survive nursing school, and you've learned a great deal about landing your first job as a nurse. This next section is to provide you a completely unbiased view of what a day in the life of a nurse truly entails. While there is certainly no "typical" day as a nurse, there are many days where you see things that you've never seen before and you have to react in ways you've never reacted before.

The beauty of being a nurse is that no two days in your career will ever be the same, and each and every day, I can make one promise to you: You WILL be challenged! Many people in other professions claim they're unhappy after a number of years, which is most likely attributed to the lack of being challenged. That is why it's important to take continuing education courses or perhaps return to school for an advanced degree in nursing. This helps in staying abreast of nursing hot topics and new and innovative ideas developing in the profession.

As a nurse, you will help people. You will touch

people's lives. You will facilitate someone's healing. You will save someone's life. You will be exposed to real-life situations that you couldn't have even fathomed before you took this job. The trick is to make sure that you can effectively deal with those challenges to ensure that you come out ahead each time. Your career will throw curveballs at you; you just need to be prepared for them. You will learn to roll with the punches.

Although almost all registered nurses have a different account of what an average day in the life of a nurse is really like, there is certainly one thing that we can all agree on: No day is going to be slow. Very few times, as a nurse, is a day slow and uneventful. This is especially true if you're working in a fast-paced environment such as the Emergency Room, for instance. Some nurses feel like their role is one that is undefined. For example, they may be called a nurse, but they are much more than that. They are the therapist, the doctor, the caretaker, the mentor, the plumber (as nurses, we laugh about this one) and the one that is ultimately responsible for nursing the patient back to health.

An important tip and worth mentioning: You should know and understand your patient's diagnosis and treatment plans and care because there is more than just a slight chance you're going to have to end up explaining everything the doctor said to the patient, soon after he leaves the room. As discussed, doctors are very brief with their patients. While some of them have better bedside manner than their counterparts, there are very few doctors who spend enough time with their patients for them to ask them all of their questions and express their concerns. In addition, many people simply do not feel comfortable expressing all of their concerns with the doctor because they feel intimidated by the doctor's presence.

CHAPTER 10

Ethics in nursing

Let's face it: We've all faced ethical and moral situations in our lives where we weren't sure of what to do or how to handle them. Some of us have faced these situations in our personal lives, but there are also many of us that have faced these situations in our professional lives as well. When ethical dilemmas enter our professional lives, things become even more complicated. All of us handle the stress and pressure of these dilemmas differently, but they certainly do affect all of us from time to time.

Unfortunately, nursing is one of those professions where the notion of facing many ethical dilemmas throughout your career is going to become more of a reality than you may think. Some nurses face ethical dilemmas on a daily basis. Why, you ask? Well, it's quite simple, really. Nursing involves dealing with a patient's health and quality of life; therefore, ethical dilemmas arise much more often in the field of nursing than they do in other professions.

PROFESSIONAL OBLIGATIONS

Patients trust that their nurses are competent in their practice, and that must show at all times. In essence, this means that nurses must be compliant with board of nursing standards and they must complete necessary continuing education requirements to demonstrate their competency.

A good rule of thumb that I sometimes tell my students is to treat your patients like you would want to be treated, or how you want a family member or friend treated if care is warranted.

CHAPTER 11

Career paths in nursing

As we mentioned before, there is no standard linear path in the nursing field. Some nurses decide to specialize when they're still in nursing school, but the vast majority of students do not know which areas of medicine they want to go into while they're still in school; therefore, many of them will find their specialties after they've had more hands-on training in the hospitals.

When I think about this, I am reminded of undergraduate students contemplating choosing a college major. Attend nursing school and gain exposure into a variety of different areas of medicine. Explore. Ask questions. Talk with your peers. Talk with your professors. Do some research. There are so many options and resources available to you, and those options are always increasing over time.

HOT, HOT, HOT CAREER CHOICES

There is no doubt that in today's contemporary society, there are some nursing fields that are hotter than fire. That being said, there is one thing I want to make crystal clear. What you choose to specialize in is your decision and yours alone, and I am not trying to persuade you in any way, but it's only fair that I let you in on what high demand specializations are currently sweeping the market. Throughout the course of my career, I have met nurses who have worked many years gaining experience and developing their skills, who later enhanced their careers in nursing by becoming nurse practitioners, nurse anesthetists, and informatics nurses. So as you can see, nursing is a broad profession of career choices. Nursing careers have been promising for decades and employment rates are expected to rise between 18% and 25% between 2011 and 2018, according to the U.S. Bureau of Labor Statistics.

Because of this information and the slow state of the economy, nursing school enrollments are up for anyone contemplating the decision to become a nurse. Since nursing has always been a stable and safe career for most people, the fact that the industry jobs continue to be on the rise is terrific news.

MEDICAL-SURGICAL NURSE: Currently, 80% of the nursing workforce comprises of medical-surgical nursing, which is the largest specialty in nursing. A medical-surgical nurse is known to perform a number of different tasks within a hospital setting which include monitoring and caring for adult patients, assisting the doctor in surgical procedures. Like all professionals in the nursing community, medical-surgical nurses are highly respected among their peers and their patients. In my opinion, every nurse is a medical-surgical nurse. There is also a certification in this specialty, CMSRN, Certified Medical-Surgical Registered Nurse where you must first have 2,000 hours or more of medical-surgical experience under your belt and at least three years of experience, to become eligible to sit for the certification exam.

ICU: Nurses with ICU experience are in high demand. The reason for this is simple: Hospitals across the country are in constant need of quality nurses to work in ICU department, which essentially creates an increased demand for travel nurses. The ICU department isn't an easy department to work in; in fact, it can be one of the most difficult ones.

NURSE ANESTHETIST: There is one particular field

of nursing that is VERY hot right now, and is expected to grow by 22% through 2018. For a job field to grow by 22% in a mere two years is nothing shy of outstanding, thus there are many students interested in this career path. That field, as you may have guessed, is none other than as a Nurse Anesthetist. Essentially, nurse anesthetists require extensive education (beyond a bachelor degree), training, and experience.

There is an unbelievable potential for growth and the demand is sky-high. In short, a nurse anesthetist is one that administers anesthesia to surgical patients, provides care for patients in the operating room, and ultimately are a part of the thorough pre-operative and follow-up care for the outpatient procedures. Although these are only a few of their many responsibilities, this is what a nurse anesthetist does in a nutshell. As you may have imagined, breaking into this specialty requires a master's degree in nursing. After completion of the program, you are eligible to sit for the certification board exam. Once successfully passed, you're officially a nurse anesthetist! This is currently the most lucrative career path for a nurse with a median annual income of $154,390 at starting.

CLINICAL NURSE SPECIALIST: According to a recent blog by thebestschools.org, a clinical nurse specialist is one who is authorized to work with patients in a clinical setting. Essentially, these nurses are certified to diagnose and treat patients who are suffering from one or more of the "normal" health problems that people seek medical attention for. Unlike a regular RN, these nurses have the ability to prescribe medicine, which makes them much more marketable and easier to place for employment.

In order to become certified, the RN degree is the first

stepping stone. After finishing your RN degree, you'll also need a bachelor's and master's degree in nursing with an emphasis on clinical practice. Sound like a lot? It does take a reasonably high amount of schooling, but keep in mind that you can also work while you attend graduate school. Not only that, but many hospitals will even pay for a portion (or all, depending on various factors) of your tuition, provided you have been with them for some time and you plan on sticking with them for a while after finishing your degree. As I've stated, the demand is very high right now, and that demand is expected to increase by 19% through 2018. Since the profession is in such high demand, the median salary for a clinical nurse specialist was $93,901 in 2015.

ADVANCED NURSE PRACTITIONER: The family nurse practitioner is the main person who alleviates the vast majority of our aches and pains. This person is usually at the forefront of our medical contacts, and is the primary person we feel the most comfortable around and trust with personal information. Nurse practitioners are an essential part of family practice. They are very similar to doctors in the sense that they have a lot of formal education and training in medicine, yet they still have the bedside manner and compassion that made them choose the nursing field. Nurse practitioners are licensed to examine patients, diagnose illnesses, and prescribe medicine under the supervision of a doctor. The laws of nurse practitioners do vary from state to state. In some states, they are able to have their own private practice, independent of a physician. In other states, this is not allowed.

If you are interested in becoming a nurse practitioner, I would encourage you to check the laws of your respective state, or any other areas of the country that you plan on possibly moving to one day, if any apply. Becoming a certified nurse practitioner is no cakewalk. First, it's required that you earn your bachelor's and master's degrees. Upon completing your master's, you can apply to receive your family practitioner certification from the American Nurses Credentialing Center of the American Academy of Nurse Practitioners. As of 2015, the median salary was $94,407, and the job market anticipates growth by 26% through the year 2020.

GERONTOLOGICAL: Gerontological nursing is an area of nursing that specializes in the care of elderly patients. This area will be in high demand now and in the future. The baby boomer population is getting "up there" in age, and the number of elderly people in the United States will soon increase, thus inflating an already large demand for nursing care by as much as 26% through the year 2020. Although this goes without saying, it's also just as important that you are patient and capable of working with the elderly on a daily basis. There are many people that want to get into this specialty, but it's not realistic for everyone.

Nurse practitioner's role involves assessing, diagnosing illnesses, creating a plan of treatment, and prescribing medications. In addition, you will also need to perform routine medical check-ups and ensure the patient is healthy and not at risk for contracting any medical problems. Getting into this field is very similar to a nurse practitioner. Essentially, you will need to have your bachelor's degree and master's degree at which time you may apply for your certification for practicing gerontology from the American Nurses Credentialing Center of the American Academy of Nurse Practitioners. Luckily, this field is a hot one. The median salary is currently $92,170, which will only increase in the next five years to perhaps a six-figure income.

NURSE EDUCATOR: I have often said that one of the greatest joys in life is working with nursing students. Since I am an adjunct nursing professor, the opportunity to work with fresh-minded students each day and teach them the skills of what nursing is all about gives me joy. The nurse educator role is one of high demand for its specialty. A survey in 2010 discovered that 56% of nursing schools in the United States were looking for nursing educators to fill open positions at their respective schools. Unfortunately, there is such a wait list to start in a nursing program, because of the shortage of nurse educators. To be eligible to become a nurse educator, one must first hold a master's degree in nursing. In addition, it is recommended you must be a certified in a specialty area. While some educators do, indeed, hold doctoral degrees, it is not necessary but this will soon change, as some states have already begun requiring a doctorate degree to teach. As for job growth, the demand for nurse educator positions is expected to exceed the national postsecondary teachers' estimate of 17% by the year 2020. The median income for a nurse educator was $83,846 in 2015 for full-time faculty members.

NURSE INFORMATICS: Nurses who specialize in nursing informatics will possess combined skills in the health informatics sector, in health science, computer science, and information technology to help healthcare providers store, retrieve, and utilize large amounts of data as it applies to patient care. The nursing informatics professional also simplifies documentation of patient care and enters patient notes using computers, mobile devices, and voice recognition software. This area of nursing professionals aims to improve the accuracy of patient data and enable critical data analysis to improve efficiency of overall patient care. Nurse informaticists have a median annual salary of $93,000, with the average being $100,717 annually.

·

So, there you have it, folks. This information is meant to illustrate the fact that there are all kinds of areas that you can specialize in and make a career out of. There are many, many different paths that you can take to become a nurse, and certainly, there is no such thing as a one-size-fits-all model. Most nursing students are very similar to most college students in the fact that they don't know what they want to "major" in or specialize in. It's hard to make such large decisions when you're young and inexperienced; luckily, the nursing profession is very forgiving since the first requirements are to obtain your degree and then you can always go back and specialize once you've been exposed to more areas of medicine that closely match your skills and interests.

CHAPTER 12

Advice from the experts

If you could offer advice to anyone thinking about attending nursing school, what would you say?

One of the best and smartest things that any nursing student can ever do is to speak with seasoned nurses who have been practicing in the field for a number of years. Nurses with a few years under their belt are truly excellent resources in order to give information, career advice, or general guidance in order to help a younger nursing student with their career. When gathering research for this book, I surveyed many of my students in an effort to find out the most valuable information that they would share with someone thinking of attending nursing school.

Myia T, stated: *"It will be challenging but you can do it. Stay positive and prayerful."*
Myia T, RN, 2011 graduate

This is excellent advice, and I know this to be true. Nursing school is challenging, but you should never let the fear of a challenge deter you from attending nursing school and reaching your true potential. If you stay positive and work hard, there is little doubt that you will succeed, as working hard and staying positive is a recipe for success in my eyes.

Edyta states: *"You must truly know in your heart and soul that this is what you want to do in your life, then you will receive a strength and help from above to conquer all. You must believe in yourself and never give up, times will be very challenging but you can do it."*

Edyta is correct. Having the dream at the core of your

heart and soul is integral, as you will then be able to find the strength within yourself to overcome adversity and all other challenges that will come your way throughout the process. Remember that no "easy" path in life is ever worth taking, and nursing is no exception.

Another critical component to surviving nursing school is to not get discouraged by others, as there are always negative people and naysayers in your life that will try and talk you out of doing the very things that your heart wants you to do. If nursing is in your heart, then there isn't a single person in the world who can take that away from you, or deter you from succeeding.

Megan M., said it best when she said: *"I would say do not get discouraged by what others say. I remember when I told people I was going back to nursing school all I heard was how hard it was, how I wouldn't have a life, how much stress it causes, and while yes, at times those may be true, it doesn't last forever! I can't believe I am three months away from obtaining my BSN. Looking back at the struggles and the weekends I missed, I still would go back and do it again because it's what I love, and in the end that's all that matters!"*
Megan M., RN, 2015 graduate

This is excellent advice because it takes all of the negativity that people say about the rigors of nursing school and it silences those concerns through passion, and the pursuit of education and an excellent career. Earlier in this book, I spoke heavily about the cost of nursing school and stated how important it was for you to be prepared for this, as some people find themselves buried in more stress over the cost of school than they do the schoolwork itself. This is problematic, as nursing school is quite expensive. The best thing you can do is to read about the cost of nursing school, student loans, and how to minimize your debt.

"Be prepared mentally and financially with a great supportive network to assist during challenging moments."
Modestine, RN, 2015 graduate

This is excellent advice, as having a strong network of family, friends, and your peers is vital in helping you overcome some of the largest challenges that you'll be facing during your time in nursing school, and even with your career as a nurse.

Another excellent bit of information is to always give it your all. While some people may think this is obvious, the unfortunate reality is that too many people enroll in nursing school and don't give it their all simply because they're too lazy, or because they have other social engagements or obligations that are preventing them from giving their full focus and attention to their academic work.

"If you decide to go to nursing school, make sure to give it your all. I saw many of my classmates in the beginning try to get by without reading or studying and it does not work that way. Many of them either had to change those habits, or they did not make it through the program. It is difficult, but I can honestly say completing nursing school and becoming a nurse, has been the most rewarding experience that I have had in life so far."
Deanna B., RN, BSN, 2015 graduate

This is quite true. I cannot convey exactly how rewarding it felt when I was wearing my cap and gown and my name was called to come up to the podium and receive my degree. Only you can experience this because only you are in control of your destiny.

More advice from the experts comes in the form of receiving help from tutors along the way.

"1) Find tutors for all classes that took the class already. [It] really helps for them to give you a heads up for the class.
2) Do 250 NCLEX questions (whatever pertains to the exam) before taking an exam. VERY IMPORTANT!!!
3) When studying mostly focus on nursing interventions and make note cards out of all of them."
Lisa B., RN, 2015 graduate

•

This invaluable information comes as no surprise. As for tutors, there is assistance available at almost all nursing schools; you just need to reach out for help if you need it. The professors in nursing school are quite helpful, and so are the tutors, and even your peers. Also, it's not just the act of studying that is so important, it's knowing how to study in order to maximize the knowledge that you've learned so that way you can earn the best score possible on the exams. Nursing school is very competitive, thus scoring the highest that you can on the exams is crucial to remaining competitive with your fellow classmates.

Please take some time to re-read and to analyze the comments from above. They are from people who have traveled the road that you want to take; therefore, their advice, guidance, and wisdom is crucial for your success. Not all of their advice may make sense to you at the moment.

Some of it may take some time to sink in, and some of it may only sink in after you're in nursing school so you can really see what they are talking about.

CHAPTER 13

Closing arguments

First off, congratulations on making it to the end of this book! Hopefully, by this point, you have a thorough understanding of what will be required of you if you decide to enroll in nursing school, as well as how the job market is going to be, and what to expect when you enter the nursing profession upon your graduation. At this time, you should be able to confidently look into the mirror and say to yourself, "I want to go to nursing school and become a nurse. After reading this book and being informed of what the nursing industry is really like, I can say with full confidence that is something I want to pursue."

If you cannot say that at this time after all that you've read and been taught throughout the course of this book, it's quite possible that there may be another field better suited for you. The purpose of this was not to persuade you to become a nurse; rather, it was meant to give you the basics of nursing — the true meaning of becoming a nurse.

Also, to put away any common stereotypes and misconceptions there are about the nursing profession and to give you the real, accurate picture from the experts in the profession. As previously mentioned, there are many, many stereotypes that surround the nursing industry and quite frankly, I have seen far too many students enter the nursing field because of what a certain movie or television show made the career look like. Needless to say, those depictions are just entertainment.

- Nursing is more than a career. It's a profession. If you don't have the passion and drive, then I would suggest against becoming a nurse, particularly if you are not ready.

• You will never be the same person again once you make the decision to enroll in nursing school. Let me clarify that. What I mean in this instance is that there are things you see and experience as a nurse that no one else in your life who is not a nurse will be able to relate to. That makes you different, but in a good way.

• You will often times be asked to play "doctor" around your friends and family. Essentially, this means that even though you may be off the clock, there's a good chance that when a friend or family member isn't feeling well or has a medical-related question, you will often bc the first person they speak with, most times even before they go to a doctor. Even after they do physically see their doctor, they often may ask you for a second opinion, and if you agree with their diagnosis and course of treatment. I usually feel flattered by these requests, and I am always happy to help. Since nursing is such a passion of mine, I certainly don't mind helping friends and family members during their time of health needs.

•

After all that has been said throughout this book, it is my sincere hope that you thoroughly enjoyed reading this book as much as I have enjoyed writing it. This project was a wonderful opportunity for me to utilize my 20 years of experience and share that information with you. My motivation for writing this book is what carried me through the process, and I am so pleased to have completed this. With the newfound knowledge you now have, take a moment to reflect on everything that you've read here. Deep down inside, you know if this is right for you, and if the dream is in your heart, there isn't a single person or event that can stop you from accomplishing your goal of becoming a nurse. I am honored to have provided you with the knowledge base you now possess. It's all yours from here, folks!

"Just found out I passed! There were three questions that I answered using what you taught me, nothing I read in any of my books about them at all. Again, thank you!"
Modestine N., BSN, RN, 2015

ABOUT THE AUTHOR

Yalanda D. Comeaux, a seasoned expert in the field of nursing, started her nursing career as an ADN (Associate Degree) nurse. She currently holds a Master's in Nursing with a focus on Education degree.

She has more than 20 years of nursing experience with 30 years in the healthcare industry. During this time she has worked in various capacities in nursing from clinical nurse, management, and nursing education with the majority her nursing background concentrated in the area of fast-paced environments like Post Anesthesia Care Unit (PACU) nursing, where she currently works as a clinical nurse. She also has work experience in areas of Critical Care (ICU), and Medical-Surgical nursing.

She is an adjunct faculty member for a School Of Nursing (SON) in the Chicago area, teaching Medical-Surgical nursing to BSN and ABSN students in a clinical setting; and she is a CMSRN, Certified Medical-Surgical Registered Nurse.

The author also holds a Master of Jurisprudence (MJ) in Health Law and Policy from Loyola University School of Law, Chicago.

She enjoys reading, traveling abroad, watching and playing tennis, and being a foodie. She is married and resides with her husband near Chicago.

The author loves to hear from readers. Connect with her in the following ways:
- Send her an email to Yalanda@RNBound.com
- Follow her on Twitter @NurseGuide_yc
- Snail mail her at:

RNBound
c/o Yalanda Comeaux
PO Box 5193
Lansing, IL 60438

Yalanda can also be heard on HUR_Voices Sirius XM channel 141 with the Traveling Culturati as the healthcare correspondent delivering tips on "Staying Healthy While Traveling."

WANT TO INVITE YALANDA TO SPEAK AT YOUR EVENT?

Send an email to Yalanda@RNBound.com, sharing details about your event, including event type, date, time, and location. If the event has a website, please let her know. Also include what you would like her to discuss at the event and any other relevant event details. Someone will get back to you within 48 hours with more booking information, including fee and availability.

NOTES

NOTES

NOTES

NOTES

NOTES